DON'T WORRY!

A SELF HELP GUIDE TO MANAGING STRESS & TENSION
Robert Poyton

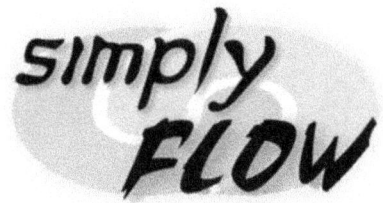

Copyright@ 2020 R Poyton

All rights reserved

The moral right of the author has been asserted

No part of this book may be reproduced in any form or by any
electronic or mechanical means including information storage
and retrieval systems, without permission in writing from the author.
The only exception is by a reviewer, who may quote short
excerpts in a review.

The author and publisher take no responsibility for any illness or
injury resulting from practicing the exercises described in this book.
Always consult your Doctor prior to training or if you have any medical issues.

Published by Cutting Edge

ISBN: 978-1-64826-143-5

"When I look back on all these worries, I remember the story of the old man who said on his deathbed that he had had a lot of trouble in his life, most of which had never happened."

- Winston Churchill

TITLES IN THE SIMPLY FLOW SERIES

Fitness Over 40

The Eight Brocades Qigong

Don't Worry!

www.simplyflow.co.uk

CONTENTS

CHAPTER ONE: INTRODUCTION
Introduction 8
Background 11
How to use this book 13

CHAPTER TWO: WHAT IS STRESS?
Stress Occurrences 17
Adrenaline Dump 18
Effects of Stress 23
Stress Triggers 24
Keeping a Journal 34

CHAPTER THREE: BREATHING
Breathing Exercises 39
Breath Shapes 42

CHAPTER FOUR: EMOTIONAL TENSION
Brain States 47
Quiet Sitting 48
Thought Control 50
Mindfulness 53
Visualisation 55
General Mindset 58

CHAPTER FIVE: PHYSICAL TENSION
Selective Tension 69
Movement 72
Massage 78

CHAPTER SIX: LIFESTYLE STRATEGIES
Compensation Activities 87
Coping Mechanisms 89
Time Management 90
Learning to Say No 94
Positive Thinking 89

Sleep 100
Diet 104
Work/Life Balance 109

CHAPTER SEVEN: PAIN & GRIEF
Pain Control 115
Coping With Grief 120
Emotional Release 121

CHAPTER EIGHT: CONFLICT & FEAR CONTROL
Conflict Resolution 127
Stress Indicators 128
Establishing Rapport 131
Fear Control 134
Fear Inoculation Stages 138

CHAPTER NINE: GOING DEEPER
Maslow's Hierarchy of Needs 143
Lifestyle Review 146
Activities & Therapies 149
Pulse Breathing 154
Extended Sitting 156
Mindful Movement 157

CHAPTER TEN: CONCLUSIONS
Stress Management Checklist 163

APPENDIX ONE
MP3 Downloads 165

APPENDIX TWO
Resources 167

APPENDIX THREE
Contact Details 169

CHAPTER ONE
INTRODUCTION

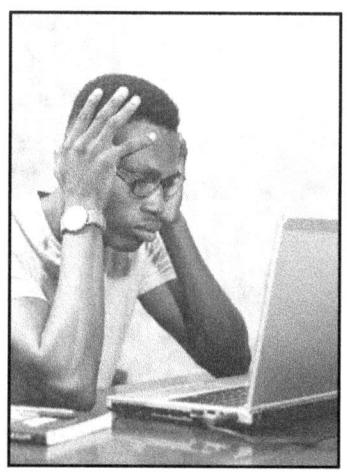

The alarm didn't go off, so you are running late for work. Get the kids sorted, and away to school. The phone rings as you are getting ready - another insurance cold call! Answering that means your toast is now burnt. Never mind, you'll pick up something on the way. A fast walk to the station, grab an overpriced sandwich at the kiosk, wolf it down on the platform.

Delays again, your train is 15 minutes late. Run into the office at the other end, you are out of breath, sweaty and annoyed and the day hasn't even started yet. There's a message on your desk, the boss wants to see you…

I'm not saying this is a typical day but, let's face it, we've all had days like it. Sometimes the world seems to be conspiring against us, we are frustrated at every turn. Yet if we live in what may be termed the First World, why should we have anything to worry about? Clean water comes out of the tap, most of us have a roof over our heads, access to technology that was unheard of even a generation ago. We have all types of entertainment on demand, you can buy almost any type of food you like at the local supermarket.

We don't have to fight off invaders, we don't have to suffer terribly from even minor ailments, or worry about being executed for our beliefs. For the most part, we live out our lives in what is, for some of the world at least, the "best time" to be alive. And the future promises even more - cures for disease, the prospect of extended life span, even great levels of tech and so on.

And yet, stress and stress-related conditions show no signs of abating. In fact, they may even be on the increase. A 2018 Gallup poll found that the majority of Americans (55%) said they had experienced stress during a lot of the day. Nearly half (45%) said they felt worried a lot and more than one in five (22%) said they felt anger a lot. This, in the richest country in the world. A similar, global poll found that levels of stress were at a new high, while levels of worry and sadness also increased.

Even more alarming, a 2018 survey commissioned in the UK by the Mental Health Foundation, found the following:

74% of UK adults have felt so stressed at some point over the last year they felt overwhelmed or unable to cope.

81% of women said this compared to 67 percent of men.

83% of 18-24 year-olds said this compared to 65% of people aged 55 and over.

32% of adults said they had experienced suicidal feelings as a result of stress.

16% of adults said they had self-harmed as a result of stress.

Why should this be? Why should people living in the relative comfort of a modern, industrialised society, feel so stressed? There are some

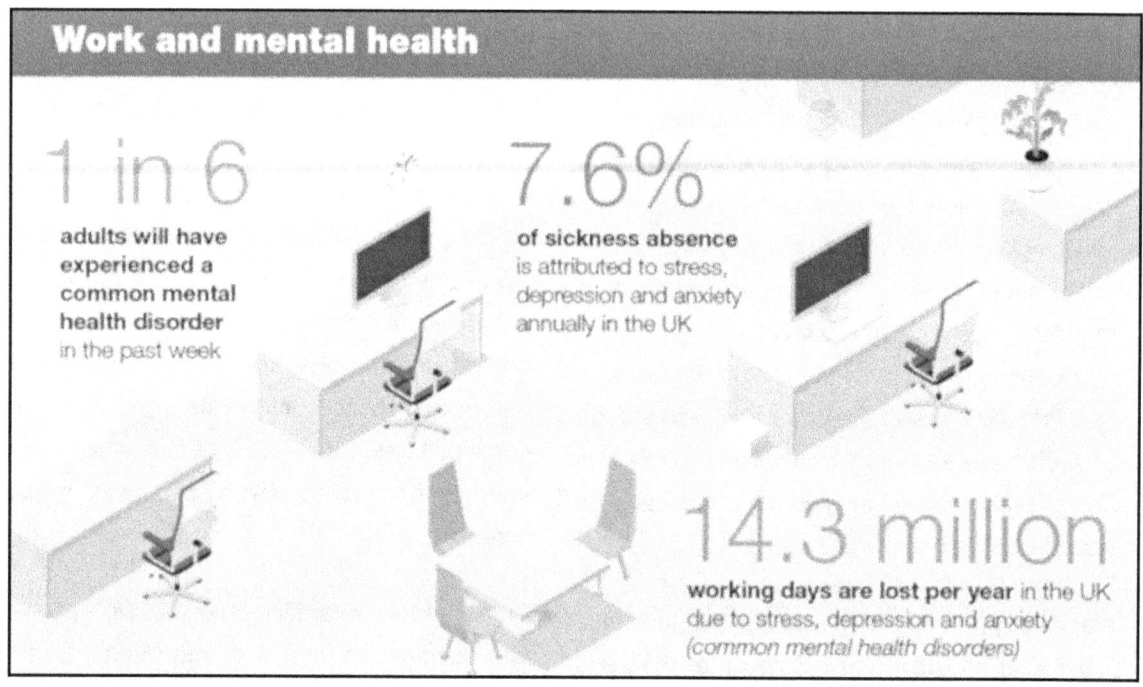

universal factors, of course. Wherever we live, as humans, we face the same issues - ageing, illness, disease and death. Then there are the social issues that also apply across the board - acceptance by our peers, relationship issues, loneliness and so on. But why should people not facing a daily struggle to survive be so stressed?

I believe the answer to that lies partly in the structure of our society and the expectations and pressures that structure brings - the pressures that, often, we put ourselves under. Add to that the huge and sudden explosion in influence of social media and other technology in our lives, as well as increasing economic and environmental uncertainty and you have more factors that contribute to increased stress levels.

To counter the gloom, it should also be recognised that mental health issues are discussed much more openly these days. In that sense, a sudden increase in mental health issues may also be a reflection of the wider acceptance and improved treatments for such issues.

It is easy to dismiss many modern concerns as just *first world issues*. After all, it's not as if we have to hunt and face dangerous predators in order to get our weekly shop! However, that dismissal would be a mistake. However facile seeming its causes, stress is very real to those who suffer from it.

We must recognise that exposure to constant even low level stress has an extremely deleterious effect on our immune system and overall well-being. In fact, it is that constant ow-level exposure that causes most of the problems.

An immediate serious threat provokes a state commonly known as *flight or fight*. In our "natural" world, the situation would likely be resolved there and then. In modern times, such as in our opening scenario, it is less easy to *fight or flight*. The stress is low level but on-going. It comes at us from many sources and all angles and is insidious. We may not even be aware that our stress levels are so high. Even worse, some regard high stress levels as a sign of success! You are actually "making it" if you live a hi-stress, hi-energy lifestyle, if you take part in "insanity" workouts, if you constantly push, compete and "win."

My aim in writing this book, is to give you an easy-to-implement self-help guide to managing everyday stress and tension. Hopefully, you will become more aware of your stress triggers and how to deal with them. There are simple strategies we can put in place to protect ourselves from incoming stress, most requiring little more than a slight shift in our outlook.

Alongside that, there are some physical activities that should mitigate the worst effects of stress on our systems. Once again these are quite simple, mostly revolving around breathing, plus a little movement. If you are interested in going deeper into healthy exercise methods, I recommend you check out our other titles for guidance.

BACKGROUND

So who am I and what is my background in this field? Well, at time of writing I'm a mid-50s man, born and raised in London, in what you would call a typical upbringing. I've experienced the same stresses as anyone else of my place and age - relationships, money worries, pressure of work (or no work at all!), death of family and friends, threats of violence, social pressures and all those things that a part of life's rich tapestry.

I should add that these are just the negative aspects, there have been plenty of positives, too! However, I have seen the result of unmanaged stress first hand, in terms of the suicide of a friend,as well as the effects of mental health issues.

As for my professional background, I had an early interest in martial arts. As a teenager, began a study of Chinese martial arts and associated health and philosophical systems - in particular, the "internal" arts of *Taijiquan* and *Qigong*. In the mid-1990s I set up my own school and became a full time instructor.

Around 2000, I became aware of Russian styles of training, in particular a method known as *Systema*. It is largely that art that I practice and teach today, alongside some of the methods from my earlier, Chinese training. Currently I teach in the UK and around Europe. My clients range from martial arts enthusiasts through to military / police and similar, professional dancers, people looking for general fitness and well-being and corporate and charity sector organisations.

People often wonder, what do martial arts have to do with health and well-being? The simple answer is that, in traditional societies, a warrior who was ill, physically or psychologically, was unable to fulfil his duties to protect the group. As such, powerful health and healing methods developed alongside the combative methods. Two sides of the same coin, you might say.

In the West, the increased use of firearms and the industrialisation of war lead to a falling away of tradition methods and a separation of the two aspects of training. In other cultures, there was a lot less separation, not to mention the fact that religious / spiritual practices of various groups, also became incorporated into the martial training systems.

For example, according to legend the famed Shaolin Temple *Kung-Fu* arts were originally developed by the Buddhist monk Da-mo (Bodhidarma) when he travelled from India to China in the 5th century. Likewise, Orthodox Christian monks in the Eastern tradition developed methods known as *Hesychasm*; particularly in monasteries such as Mount Athos. In brief these are methods of breathing associated with prayer and an overall "quiet" approach to life. Both of these traditions developed and intertwined alongside the warrior arts, in fact it was not uncommon for retired warriors to move into monasteries and become monks.

In modern times, scientific research has added another strand to this mix, and, even now, science is constantly "re-discovering" something that these old arts have been quietly practicing for centuries! That is not to say that there are no charlatans about. When engaging in any form of complementary medicine it is advisable to be aware of the practitioners background and qualifications. But overall, these ancient traditions a give us a rich seam to mine for modern times, be that in context of survival methods or physical / emotional /spiritual practices.

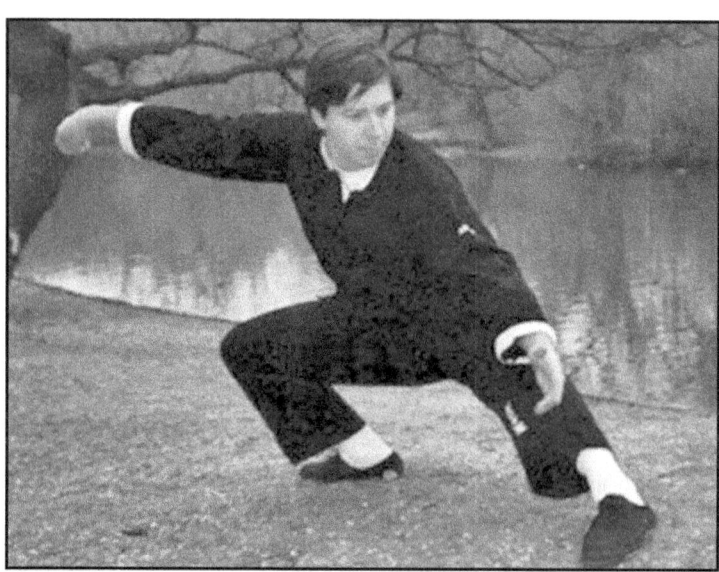

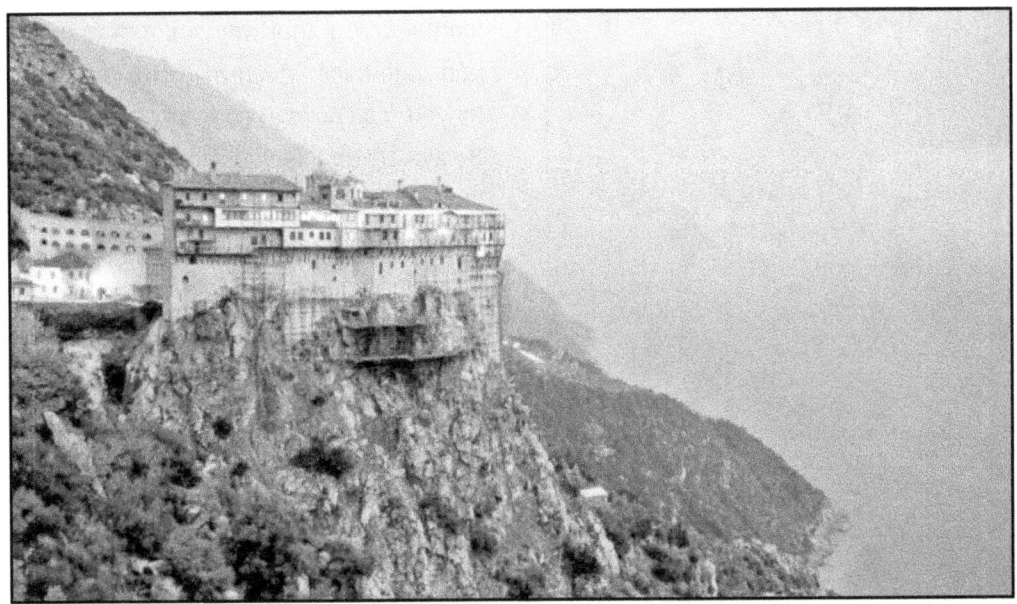

The art of Systema (the System), especially, is a modern synthesis of many older Russian traditions, passed through the filter of extensive research and field experience and application. While few of us undergo the pressures of extreme military action, the practice of Systema has considerable stress-management aspects and benefits, having been instrumental in helping many veterans with PTSD, for example.

Incidentally, I will be discussing some scientific background in this book, but will be keeping it fairly brief and basic. I want this to be a practical book rather than a theoretical one. However, the internet gives us access to much so information, so please do conduct your own research, too. I will be adding some personal experiences and anecdotes in as well, both my own and some from people close to me. Sharing our experiences is a powerful tool in dealing with stress and anxiety. If nothing else it helps us to realise we are not the only ones feeling this way!

I've mentioned the religious background to some of these practices, such as Christian, Buddhist and Taoist. I would just like to add that it is not necessary to subscribe to any particular religious or other belief in order to get benefit from these exercises. Whether or not religious faith has a part to play in your life is entirely up to you, no "belief" is required for our exercises.

HOW TO USE THIS BOOK

I suggest the best way to use this book is to give it a read through to get a grasp on the basic principles and direction. From there, try one or two of the simple exercises and work from there. We will generally be using the *Problem - Reaction - Solution* model. That means that we

Simply Flow

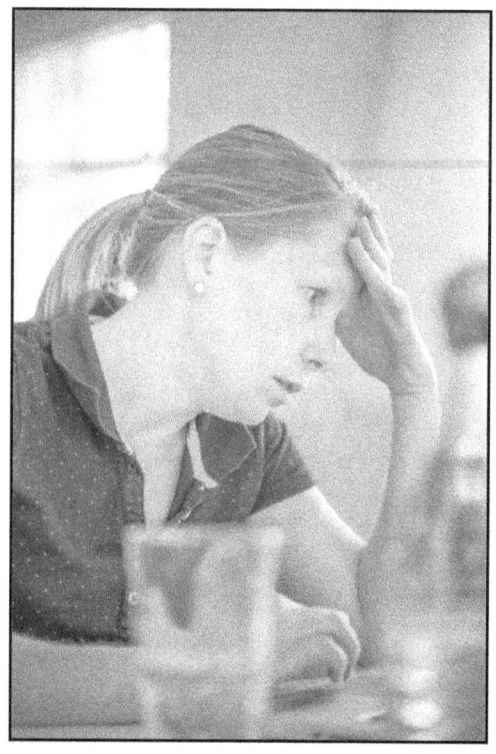

first recognise the Problem, ie the issues causing the stress. From there we talk about Reaction - what are the immediate measures we can take to mitigate the effects of stress? And following that, we move to look at a Solution. Are there steps we can take to prevent or lessen the chances of the stressful situation arising again?

Those steps may involve changes in lifestyle or, at least, in some aspects of your life. Take these things step-by-step. Don't try and implement everything at once, that may be a monumental challenge! Change is best affected in small, manageable doses. That way you can also monitor progress and tweak your approach as required. To this end, I recommend keeping a journal or log, that way you can track progress and determine which methods re working best for you. You have already taken the hardest step. By picking up this book you have acknowledged that you have stress in your life and that you are prepared to deal with it! That is a very positive action and one that gives us a solid foundation to build on.

Bear in mind that this process is not about getting rid of stress altogether - that would be impossible. Even the calmest, most serene person on the planet gets stressed at some point! The important thing is how we manage and cope with that stress. Do we control it or do we let it control us?

I would also add that if any deeper emotional or mental issues come to light during this process, you should have them addressed by a medical professional. There are many types of counselling available these days, we will discuss some of those later on. Hopefully, though, if we can nip stress in the bud, we can prevent minor issues developing into full blown conditions.

I hope this book also give you the tools to help others. A trouble shared is a trouble halved, so the old saying goes. I certainly find that increasing self awareness helps us to be more sympathetic to the troubles of others and foster an environment where issues can be talked over and positive action taken.

If, after reading the book, you have any

questions, please feel free to get in touch via our website. Please remember to always check with your medical professional before trying any type of exercise and/or if you have any deeper issues arising. In more serious situations, there are people you can speak to, details will be provided in the Appendices.

One last thing other before we start. Because of the subject, we will be addressing many of the more negative aspects of life in this book. You might, for example, read through all our examples of the issues that can cause stress and feel more depressed than when you started!

Now, we don't want to ignore the negatives, part of our stress management strategy is to bring problems out into the open. But please be aware that there are just as many positives in life to balance out the bad things!

Let us begin, then, by defining exactly what stress is, look at some of its causes and discuss the effects it can have.

.

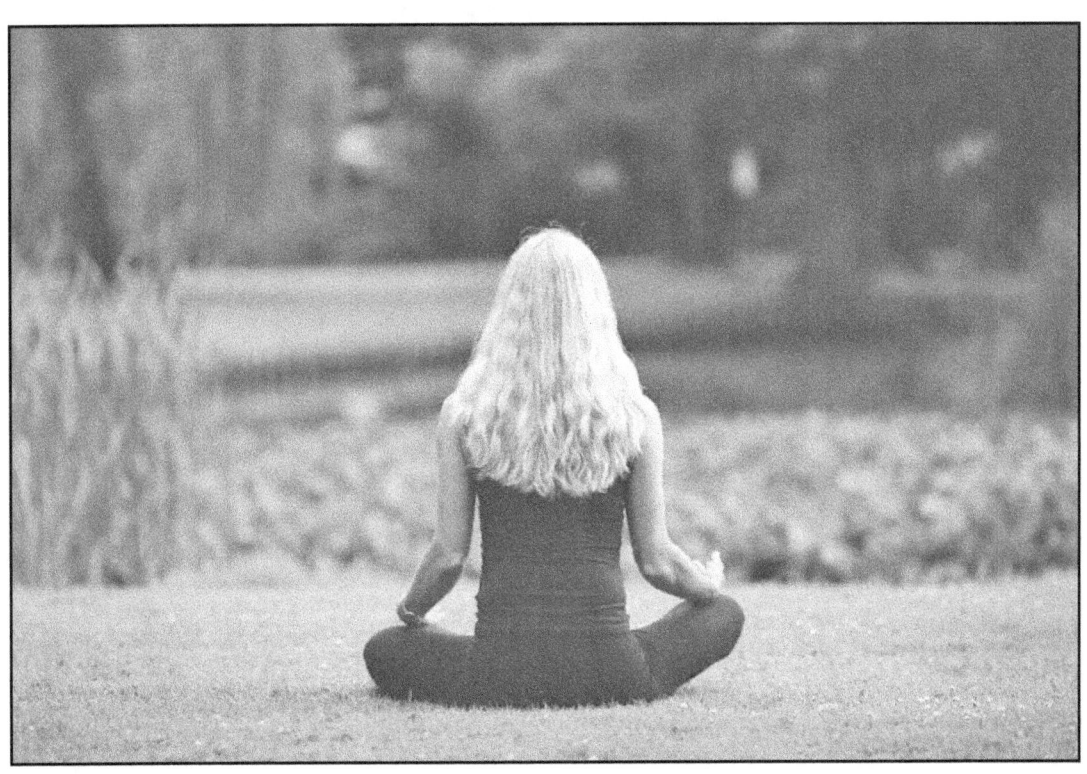

CHAPTER TWO
WHAT IS STRESS?

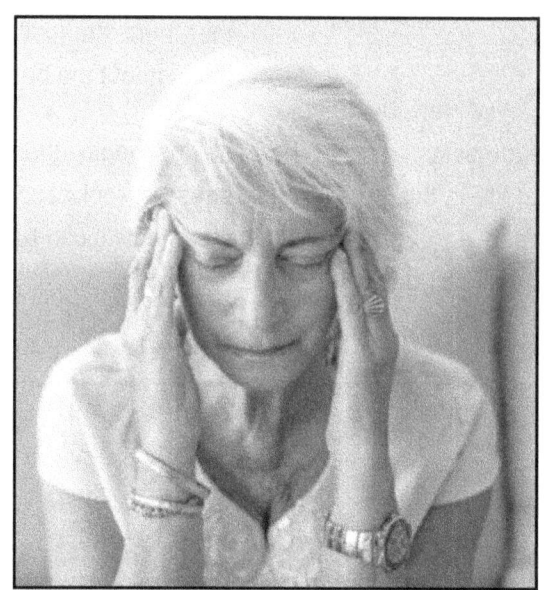

The dictionary definition of stress is: *a state of mental or emotional strain or tension resulting from adverse or demanding circumstances.*

As we know, stress can develop in many situations. It can be accumulative and it will affect us in different ways at different times in our life. No one is immune to or beyond stress. In fact, a person who seems the most bright and cheerful may be a person who is just good at hiding their stress. We can broadly divide when stress occurs into three different time frames.

STRESS OCCURRENCES

IMMEDIATE STRESS

This is the type of stress triggered by an immediate threat to our physical safety. We step out in the road and a car speeds towards us, for example. In this case, we should recognise that stress is not a bad thing, it is an indicator of danger. In such a potentially hazardous situation, our stress response kicks in and triggers what is known as our *Fight, Flight or Freeze Response* (FFFR). If all goes well, this provides our body with the necessary boost to react to the danger, to move away from it, or to confront it.

The good thing about this type of stress is that the physical action not only hopefully resolves the situation, be it to fight or flee, it also actually helps flush the chemicals produced by the *Adrenal Dump* out of the system. The situation is dealt with, and we move on.

EPISODIC STRESS

This is what we might call "everyday" stress. That may be the sort of situations from our opening scenario in the Introduction. As we mentioned before, the problem in modern times is that our FFFR is often triggered by a situation where it is not appropriate to fight or flee - dealing with a difficult client at work, perhaps. In that case, the adrenal chemicals are not flushed out of the system and, psychologically, the issue may remain unresolved, meaning we carry that stress around with us for the rest of the day.

As humans, we generally live in the past or the future. There are very few times where we actually live "in the moment." In some ways, this is a good thing. We enjoy memories, we form relationships and associations, we use our experiences to plan ahead. However, living too much in the past may mean that we "hang on" to previous bad experiences. We allow those experiences to shape our current life, we live in their shadow.

Better, if we can, to move on with our lives, free of that negativity. Now, in the case of severe trauma, that may be a difficult thing to achieve, and this is where professional counselling or similar help is invaluable. But the same principle applies even on a smaller level. Say someone cuts you up in traffic on the way to work. You can carry that anger around with you all day, or you can leave it in the car when you get out!

In the course of a day we may have several episodic stress incidents. Individually, they may not amount to much but imagine each incident is a rock. Each time you get stressed, you pick up a rock and put it in your pocket. By the end of the day you may be so weighed down you can barely move. Then you take all the rocks home and show them to your family. You may even lay awake at night counting them!

FUTURE STRESS

Living in the future means that we can plan ahead, we can look forward to events. However, it can also lead to our third form of stress - worry about things that haven't happened yet, or may not ever happen. This could be prompted by real enough concerns. *Will I be able to pay the rent next month?* It may be prompted by fear of becoming ill, or getting old. It could stem from be anticipation about a future event - an interview, for example. It may even be prompted by less personal issues - climate change, the fear of crime, a general feeling that everything is getting worse.

Research has shown that people suffering from acute anxiety orders are much more prone to live in the future. Concerns about what may or may happen overwhelm the experience of being in the now, and so prompt the same body/brain response as being in immediate danger. Of course, by their very nature, there is even less chance of resolving these issues in the here and now

THE ADRENALINE DUMP

We will next examine what happens to our body in that "immediate danger" situation. This is often called the *Fight or Flight Mechanism*, or the *Adrenaline Dump*. Strictly speaking, neither term is completely scientifically accurate, but they will do as a starting point. In fact, the latest research is suggesting that the adrenal response is actually driven by the bones. According to new studies, under stress conditions, the skeleton floods the bloodstream with the bone-derived hormone osteocalcin and it is this which triggers the FFFR. In any case, in humans we know that adrenaline is released as a result of that trigger.

Adrenaline, also called epinephrine, is a hormone released by your adrenal glands, which are situated at the top of each kidney. These glands are responsible for producing many hormones, including aldosterone, cortisol, adrenaline, and noradrenaline. They are controlled by another gland called the pituitary gland.

Adrenaline is released in response to a stressful, exciting, dangerous, or threatening situation. It helps the body to react more quickly, making the heart beat faster, increasing blood flow to the brain and muscles, and stimulating the body to make sugar to use for fuel. This sudden release is what is termed the *Adrenaline Dump*. The whole process begins in the brain. When

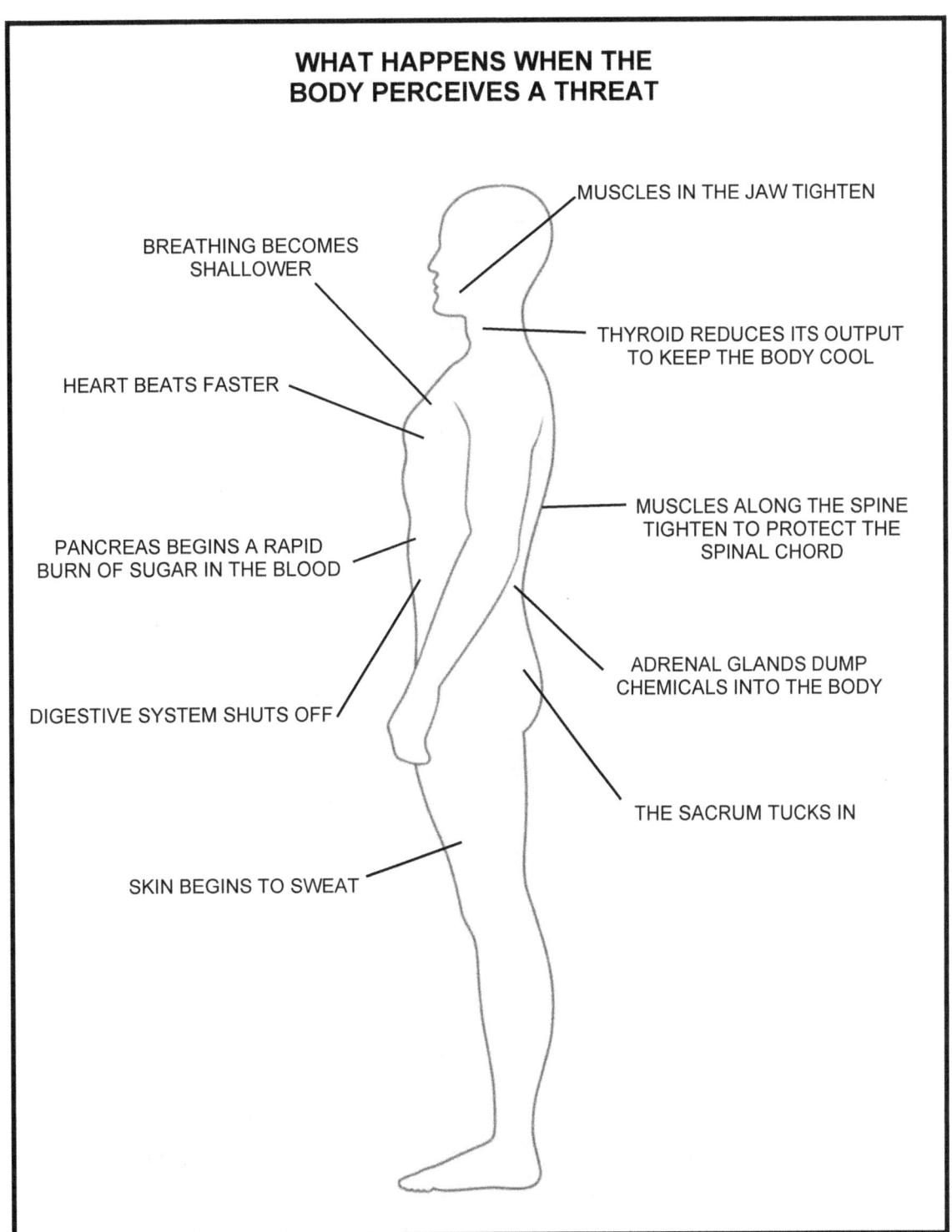

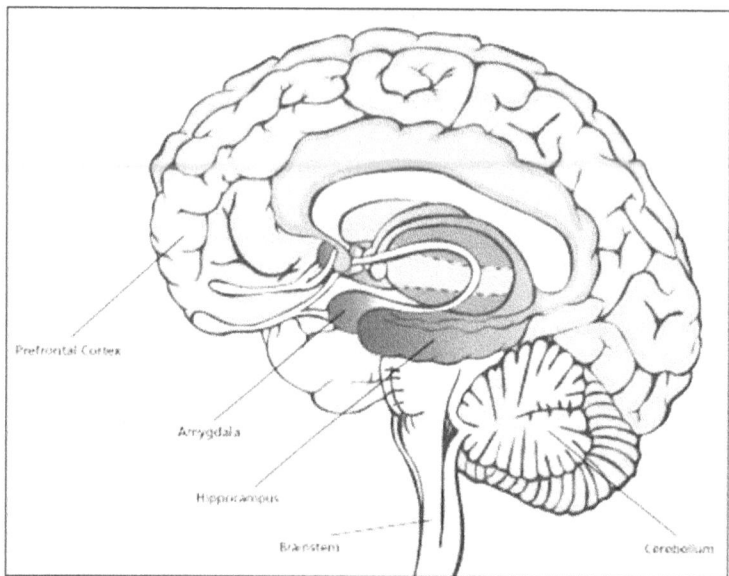

we perceive a dangerous situation, information is sent to a part of the brain called the amygdala. This is a collection of nuclei found deep within the temporal lobe. There are two amygdalae, one in each hemisphere.

The term amygdala comes from Latin for almond, so named because of the shape of the nuclei. The amygdala has important roles in emotion and behaviour, fear behaviour in particular. Information about fearful stimuli can reach the amygdala before we are even consciously aware of it. This is because a pathway runs from the thalamus to the amygdala, and sensory information about fearful stimuli is sent along this to the amygdala before it is processed by the cortex.

In other words, we can have a fear reaction before we even have time to think about it. A good example of this is a loud bang! Without thinking, we flinch and turn towards the sound.

In addition to fear response, the amygdala is also involved in forming memories associated with strongly emotional events and also plays a role in anxiety. While fear is a response to a threat that is actually present, anxiety is the worry that comes from thinking about a potential threat, one that may not even materialise. Some studies suggest that the amygdala may be overactive in people with anxiety disorders. Recent research has also found that the amygdala is also active during positive experiences. This has led researchers to somewhat review the role of the amygdala, understanding that it assigns positive value to stimuli as well as aiding in the formation of memories that have an especially strong emotional component.

So, when we are exposed to a fearful stimulus, information is immediately sent to the amygdala, which then send signals to the hypothalamus to trigger the FFFR. We can think of the hypothalamus as the command centre of the brain. It communicates with the rest of the body through the sympathetic nervous system. In our situation, the hypothalamus transmits a signal through autonomic nerves to the adrenal medulla. When the adrenal glands receive the signal, they respond by releasing adrenaline into the bloodstream. Once in the bloodstream, adrenalin:

- binds to receptors on liver cells to break down larger sugar molecules into a smaller, more readily usable sugar (glucose); this gives your muscles a boost of energy

- binds to receptors on muscle cells in the lungs, causing faster breathing

- stimulates the heart cells to beat faster

- triggers blood vessels to contract and directs blood toward the major muscle groups

- contracts muscle cells below the surface of the skin to stimulate perspiration

- binds to receptors on the pancreas to inhibit the production of insulin

These changes happen rapidly, so fast, in fact, that you might not even fully process what is happening. This rush of adrenaline is what gives you the ability to react to a threat before you've even had a chance to even think about it.

Of course, that rush may also occur in non-dangerous situations. People take part in certain activities just for the adrenaline rush. Skydiving, bungee jumping, even watching a scary movie can all trigger an adrenaline dump. There is

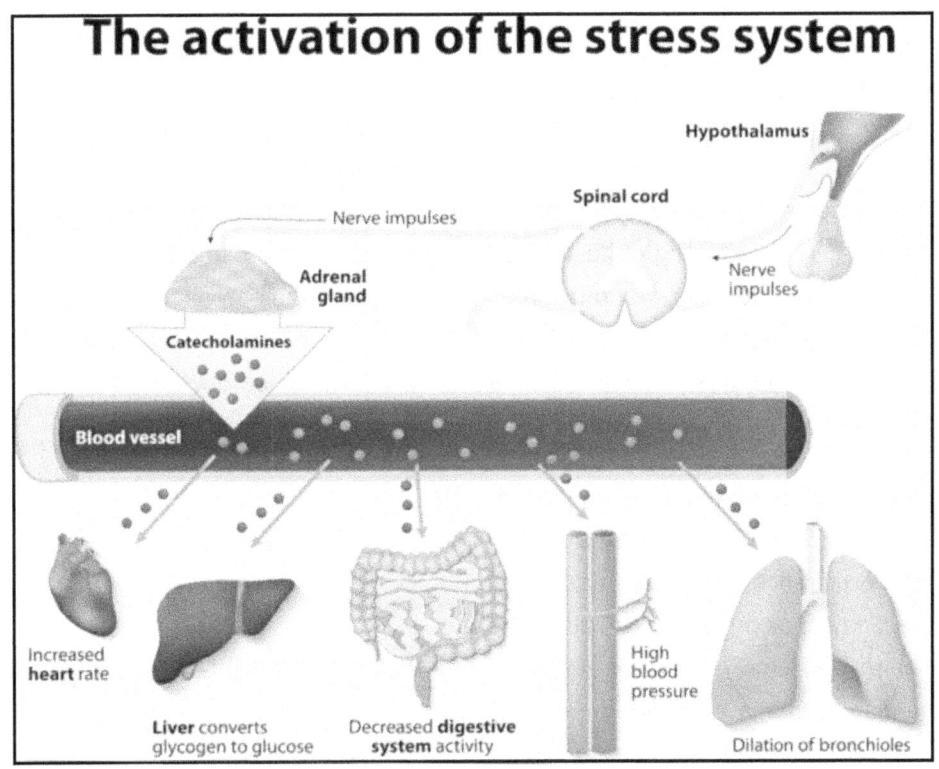

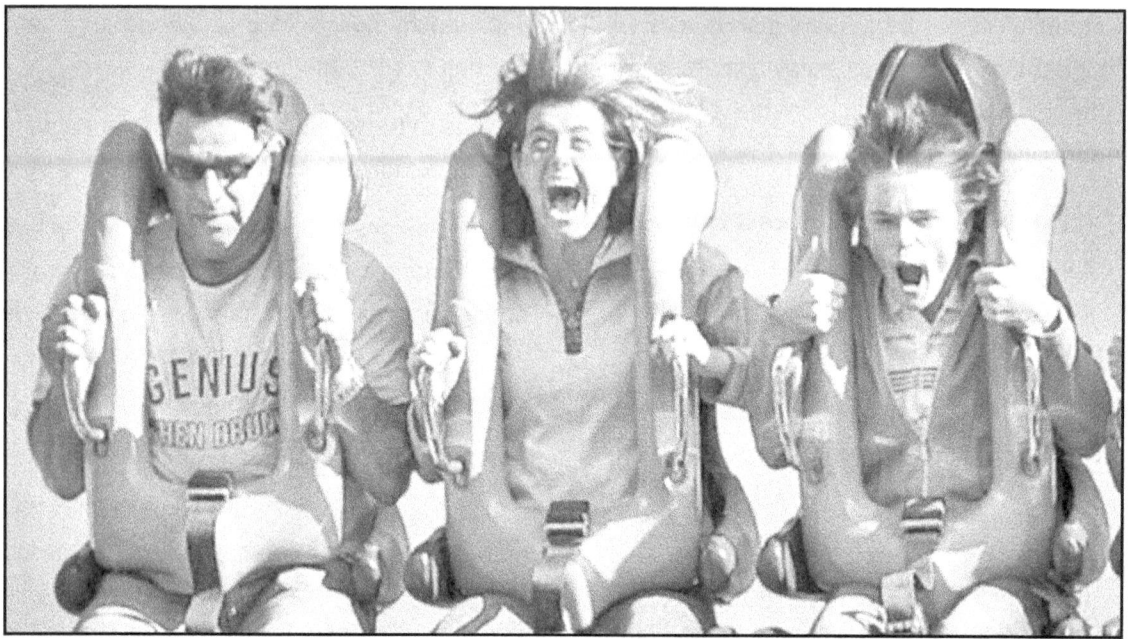

even the term "adrenaline junkie" for those who become perhaps a little too keen on the experience and are constantly seeking that boost of energy.

Along with the effects listed above, the Adrenal Dump may also give us a feeling of heightened senses, increased pain tolerance, and make us feel stronger. On the negative side, we may also become jittery and nervous, lose fine motor function and go into "tunnel vision" mode.

The effects of adrenaline can last up to an hour. It is not uncommon for people to get *the shakes* as part of that experience, or even feel nauseous. This is the body making efforts to flush the system clean. Over time, persistent surges of adrenaline can damage the blood vessels, increase blood pressure, and so increase the risk of heart attack or stroke. They can also contribute to anxiety, weight gain, headaches and insomnia.

Incidentally, although we have name-checked adrenaline here, we should not overlook the role of cortisol in this process too. In fact, cortisol is often called the "stress hormone." It is also produced in the adrenal glands and plays a part in the fight-or-flight instinct but is also involved in a number of other functions. For example, it:

- manages the use of carbohydrates, fats, and proteins

- keeps inflammation down

- regulates blood pressure

- increases blood sugar (glucose)

- controls the sleep/wake cycle

If we think of adrenaline as a short term response to danger, then cortisol is the longer term hormone. Its level is being constantly monitored by the brain. Most cells in the body have cortisol receptors, which receive and use the hormone in different ways. For instance, when your body is under stress, cortisol can alter or shut down functions that get in the way. Those might include the digestive system, the immune system, or even our growth processes.

In this sense, cortisol may be considered the more insidious of the two chemicals. A full blown adrenaline rush is hard to miss. Increased cortisol levels may not be so noticeable. In fact, if we are in a constant state of low-level stress, we may regard how we feel as being completely normal! But prolonged levels of cortisol in the bloodstream (such as those associated with chronic stress) have been shown to have many negative effects, from increased blood pressure to difficulty sleeping and more.

THE EFFECTS OF STRESS

We know that in times of stress, resources are diverted from some body systems to others. One place resources are drawn from is the immune system. The immune system is a collection of billions of cells that travel through the bloodstream. They move in and out of tissues and organs, defending the body against foreign bodies (antigens), such as bacteria, viruses and cancerous cells. The main types of immune cells are white blood cells. There are two types of them, phagocytes and lymphocytes. Stress hormones decrease the latter . The lower our lymphocyte level, the more at risk we are for viruses, such as the common cold and cold sores.

Modern research has also shown the prolonged stress alters the effectiveness of cortisol to regulate the body's inflammatory response. In effect, immune cells become insensitive to cortisol's regulatory effect. Unregulated inflammation is thought to promote the development of many diseases.

Stress responses also have an effect on the digestive system. During stress, digestion is inhibited and post-stress, digestive activity increases. This may affect the health of digestive system and cause gastric ulcers. Stress also produces an increase in blood cholesterol levels, through the action of adrenaline and noradrenaline on the release of free fatty acids. This produces a clumping together of cholesterol particles, leading to clots in the blood and in the artery walls and occlusion of the arteries. Along with this, raised heart rate is related to rapid build-up of cholesterol on artery walls. High blood pressure results in small lesions on the artery walls, and cholesterol tends to get trapped in these lesions.

Stress can also have an indirect effect on illness as it is associated with all manner of bad habits, for example smoking, drinking alcohol to excess, poor diet due to lack of time, lack of exercise for the same reason, lack of sleep etc. All these things may combine to bring lack of energy, problems with sleep, headaches, poor judgment, weight gain, depression, anxiety, and a host of other ills.

STRESS CATEGORIES & TRIGGERS

We can broadly divide stress into four categories. There is some cross-over between them, but these categories can be useful in helping us to pinpoint the type of stress and so take the appropriate measures to manage it.

Physical Stress
An immediate, physical threat (violence, an accident), strenuous activity (exercise, having to lift a heavy weight), discomfort (sitting too long in one position)

Mental Stress
Work pressures (too much work), worries (money), nerves (job interview, performance.)

Emotional Stress
Relationships difficulties, lack of relationships, sexual frustration, family pressures

Spiritual
Depression, lack of purpose, feelings of disconnection

Within the above categories, there are numerous things that can bring stress into our lives and they may affect us in different ways at different times. If things are going well, we can usually weather one or two setbacks with no problem. If things are not going so well, we may feel the effect of a particular situation or disappointment more keenly. The stress accumulates. On the other hand, we may be very successful in some areas of our life, but experience stress in others. For example we may be financially very comfortable, yet feel isolated and lonely. We may be less well off but have a great supportive network of friends and family.

It is very important to recognise our Stress Triggers. Some of these will appear quite obvious, others less so. Sometimes stress is caused by an underlying issue and brought to the surface by a totally unrelated incident. Think of the bad day you have and the last straw is a person pushing in front of you in a queue. They may well take the brunt of all your underlying stress, way out of proportion to their actual transgression!

Once we identify our Stress Triggers, we can take steps to avoid them, or at least manage exposure to them. As the old saying goes, *prevention is better than cure*. Of course, in some cases, avoiding exposure to the Stress Trigger may be very difficult, or even impossible, in which case we need to learn how to modulate our response to it.

So, let's begin an examination of potential Stress Triggers, starting with the big three!

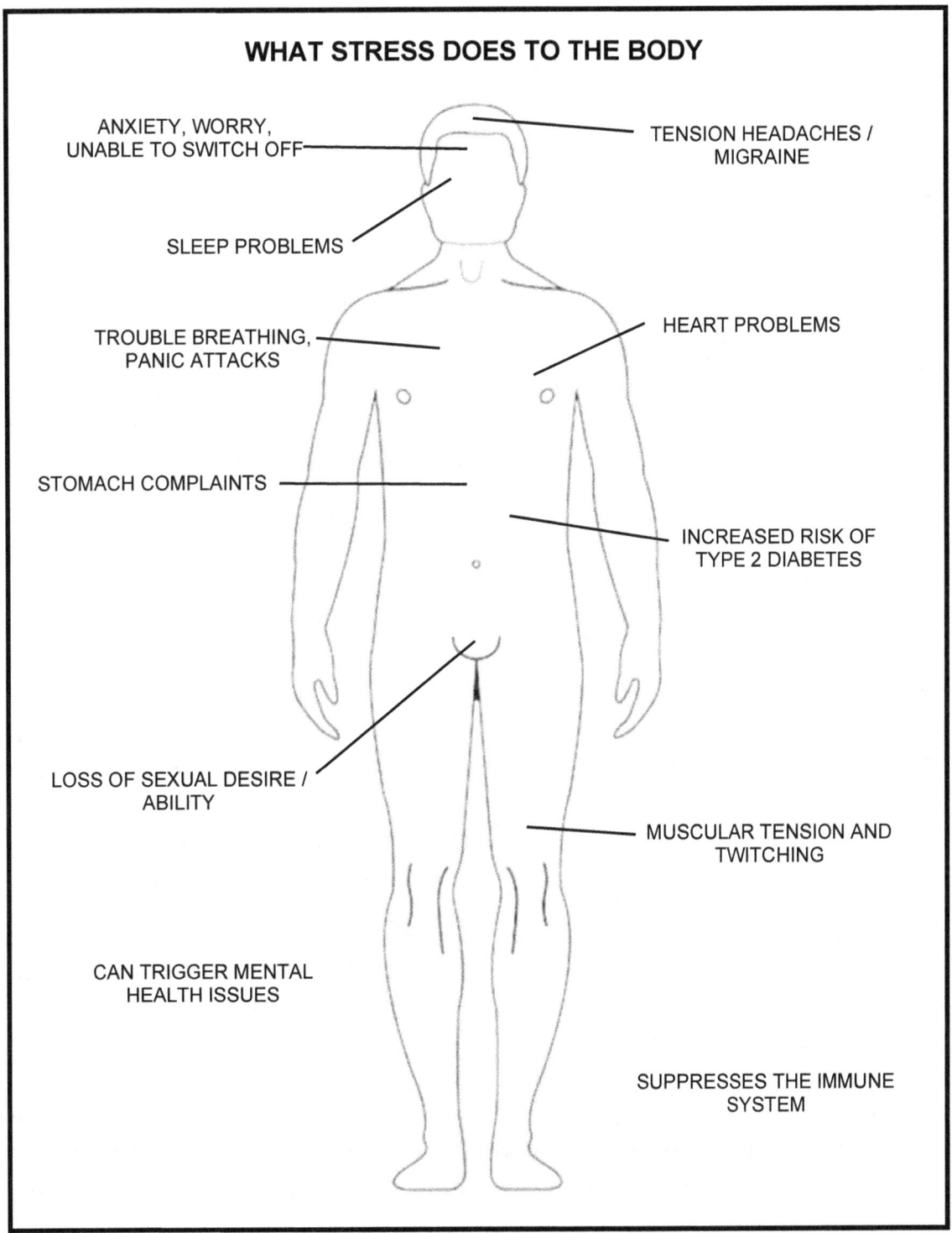

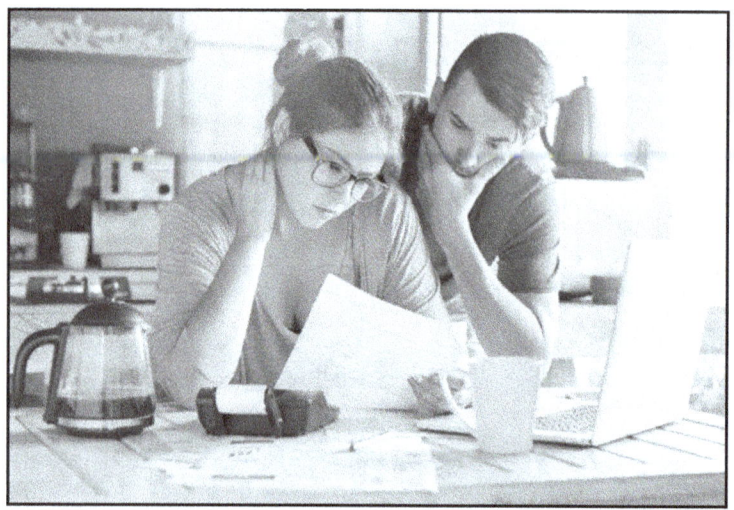

MONEY

In modern times, money usually tops the charts as the number one source of stress. On the face of it, this may seem strange. After all, if you live in the UK and earn the current average wage, you are actually amongst the top 5% most wealthy people in the world. When put into that context, why should anyone in the developed world have to worry about money?

The truth is that, whatever you think of our current economic system, we need money to survive. Unless you are lucky enough to be born into wealth, most people have to work in order to earn money to pay for housing, food, clothing and everything else that contributes to a reasonable standard of living. When income does not match outgoings, stress can result, especially if there is a significant gap. Benefits or charity may assist but relying on either of those can bring another form of stress to the situation, particularly if you have to deal with various agencies, have to wait for help, and so on.

So while incomes are relatively high in our world, so are prices and the general cost of living. I wouldn't suggest for one moment that puts anyone in the same position as a factory worker in the Far East but not begin able to adequately clothe your kids or worrying about the bills is going to cause anyone stress.

Perhaps a side issue is that our improved living standards also raise expectations. As a kid in the 1960s, we were happy at Christmas to receive a few simple gifts, some pieces of fruit and some chocolate. I recently saw what a friend was buying his son for Christmas, it included hundreds of pounds worth of electronics. Now, that may sound a bit Scrooge-like or *it weren't like that in my day!* but there is an element of truth to it nonetheless. Managing expectations, then, is one aspect of our stress management.

The stress that comes from concerns over money can be hard to avoid. This may be a case of trying our best to manage our response rather than being able to avoid it altogether. It may sound odd, but there can be stress caused by having a lot of money too. Yes, I know, we should have such a problem! Yet when we look particularly at people who have had a big win on the Lottery, not all stories have a happy ending. People in that situation may find a change in attitude from the people around them. They may feel everyone is now "just after their money" and, in some cases, they may be right! Such issues would be rare though, especially when set against the number of people who are really struggling to live and raise a family.

WORK

As we already mentioned, most of us have to work in order to make money. If we are lucky, we enjoy our job and get more from it than just money. If not, we may have another cause of stress. Work stress comes in a few forms. It could be the pressure of not having secure employment. We may be on a short term contract, the company we work for may face financial difficulties, we could be facing cuts in staff. Very few jobs seem as secure these days as they were a few decades back. Our Careers Officer at school used to advise "get a job in a bank, you'll be set for life." Well, that clearly no longer applies.

It could be that your conditions or hours of work bring stress. Working irregular shift patterns has been shown to have a negative effect on health. It may also mean you have less time to see family and friends. Perhaps the work is dangerous or unpleasant. At one time I had a job working outside. Great in summer, miserable in winter!

These factors aside, I've found that the biggest stress triggers at work are the people that you work with! The job I mentioned above was outdoors but, cold weather aside, was actually enjoyable, the team were a good laugh and we were allowed to get on with the job with a minimum of interference. I've worked in more "high-powered" companies where office politics, in-fighting, points scoring and all the rest actually made the place a misery to work, even though the actual job itself was involved and interesting.

Workplace bullying can be an issue, along with harassment, inappropriate behaviour and the like. Fortunately, such behaviour is much less

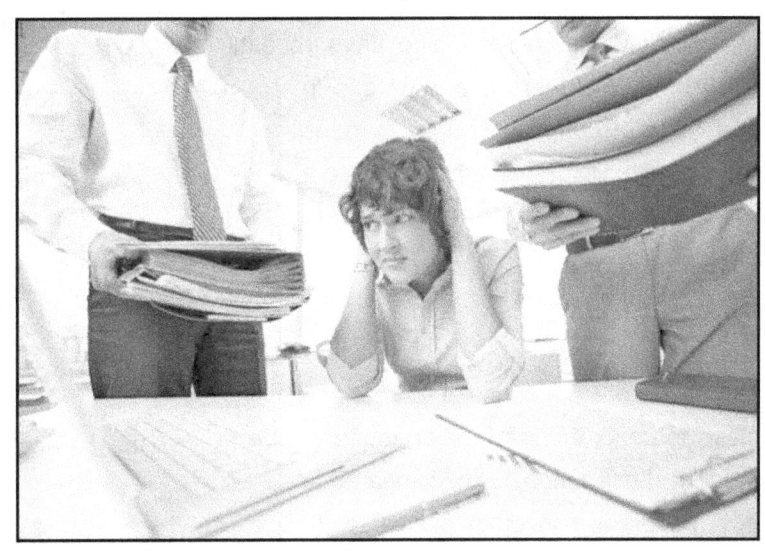

tolerated these days, though still unpleasant to experience and not always easy to confront.

Work can also bring pressure to perform, particularly where either staffing levels or competitiveness are issues. Doing more with less resources can be challenging to say the least. Likewise, having to constantly be *Salesman of the Month* or similar will bring its own pressures.

Allied to work stress is the issue of not having work. Being unemployed can also have psychological as well as financial consequences. People may feel they are of less value if they are not working, they may feel shame about being unable to provide for the families. They may feel life is lacking structure. If the issue is long term, such as a health condition, a person may feel trapped in the situation, with little prospect of change.

In a similar vein, people who have recently retired may feel there is a large gap in their lives. Routines change, there is more time to fill, perhaps they become a little isolated, there is less interaction with others.

HEALTH

Our personal state of health, or of those close to us, is the third major cause of modern stress. Once again, compared to how people live in other places, or in even relatively recent past times, we generally have it pretty good. Major diseases such as typhoid are now under control. If we get an infection, it can be easily cleared up, if we get injured, there is access to hospitals.

Having said that, we are, of course, still susceptible to all manner of ailments, not to mention possible injury. Most of us have had a shunt in the car at some point. This usually results in some minor damage to the vehicle but in serious cases can lead to life-changing injuries. With the onset of any serious illness or condition comes the question of work and care. This may be our own - we are too ill to work - or it may be another - we have to take time off work to care for a family member.

Ageing is unavoidable (I'm trying my hardest, though!) and with that come thoughts of care homes, infirmity, potential lack of income and so on. Recently highlighted are also issues such as Alzheimers, which brings us onto mental health.

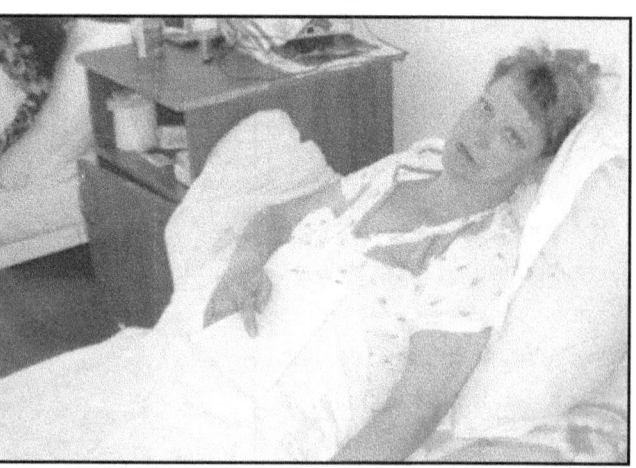

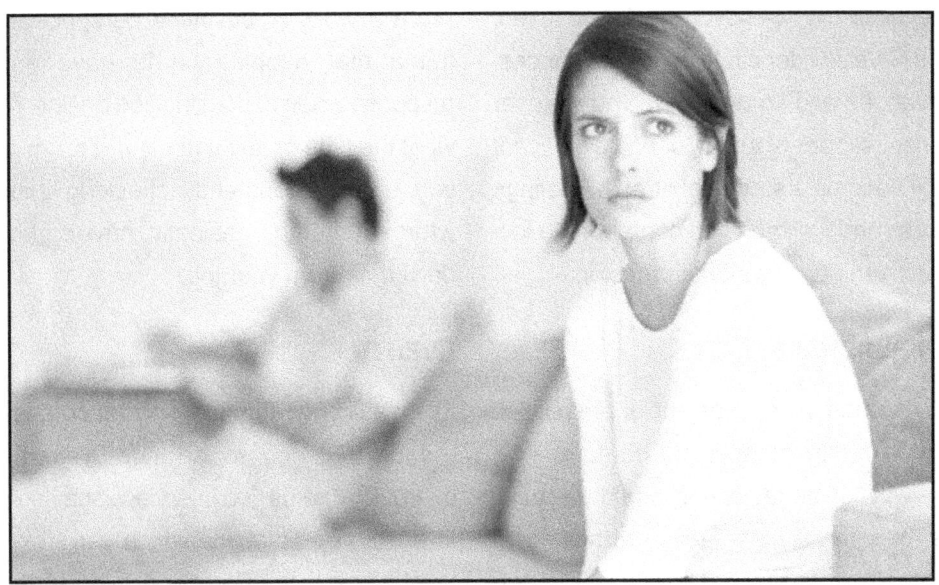

There has been much improvement in the diagnosis, care and acceptance of mental health issues in recent years. Going back even a generation we can see how people were routinely institutionalised, sometimes for their whole life, for any type of mental issue. Often, these were what be regarded today as minor conditions. There are even examples of women being institutionalised for being unmarried mothers!

Today, conditions such as depression, autism, ADHD and so on are much more likely to be recognised and appropriate treatment offered. There can still be considerable stress involved, though, both for the person and for their family. Once again, this may be an issue where stress cannot be avoided but hopefully we can do something to manage its effects

RELATIONSHIPS

We have mentioned the role of family and friends above, of course these may also be a source of stress and irritation. Family issues can range from misbehaving kids to a partner with gambling problems or having to deal with infidelity. These may be minor issues, they may go as far as being involved in an abusive relationship, whether that abuse is physical or psychological.

I doubt there is a couple anywhere that has not argued at some point and any relationship is subject to is ups and downs and disagreements. The basis for that may be financial, it may be over behaviour, or a question of roles in the relationship. Families can fall out over politics, choice of partner, lifestyle, or almost anything else!

Alongside our family, we have a social circle too. Most of us have a wider circle of acquaintances, work colleagues and so on, as well as a closer circle of friends. Lack of either, or of a *significant other*, may become a source of stress. Feelings of loneliness and isolation can contribute to low self esteem and tip over into depression.

SOCIAL PRESSURES

Alongside relationships come social pressures. This may be family pressure to conform to a particular way of behaviour, it could be peer pressure, or it might be a feeling of having to "keep up with the Joneses." Personal fulfillment, social status, a feeling of belonging are all facets of human nature. All feature in *Maslow's Hierarchy of Needs* (more of which later) and issues around them can contribute to feelings of stress and anxiety.

I think the most modern form of peer-related stress comes via social media. It is now possible to be plugged in 24/7 to the net. On the plus side, this helps us keep in touch with friends and family all round the world. On the minus side, it can also expose us to fake news, cyber-bullying, stalking or even issues around on-line addiction.

From a work or business perspective, I have found that people like to have an instant response when contacting you on-line, no matter what the time of day and night! This might mean you end up constantly checking your phone when at home, basically never getting any downtime from your job.

EVENTS

Life is full of events that can be potential stress triggers. Having to arrange a wedding, for example. Exams, job interviews, having to speak in public, all situations which can trigger some level of anxiety. The good thing is that these situations tend to be quite short term - once the event is over we can move on. However they may stack up with other triggers, especially family ones where weddings are concerned. The fallout from some weddings may last for years! Holiday times, such as Christmas, bring their own set of pressures, from financial to having to entertain a house full of relatives.

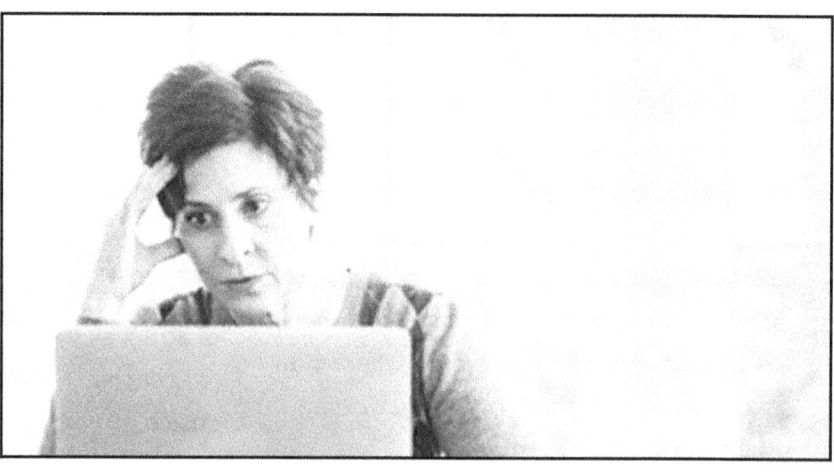

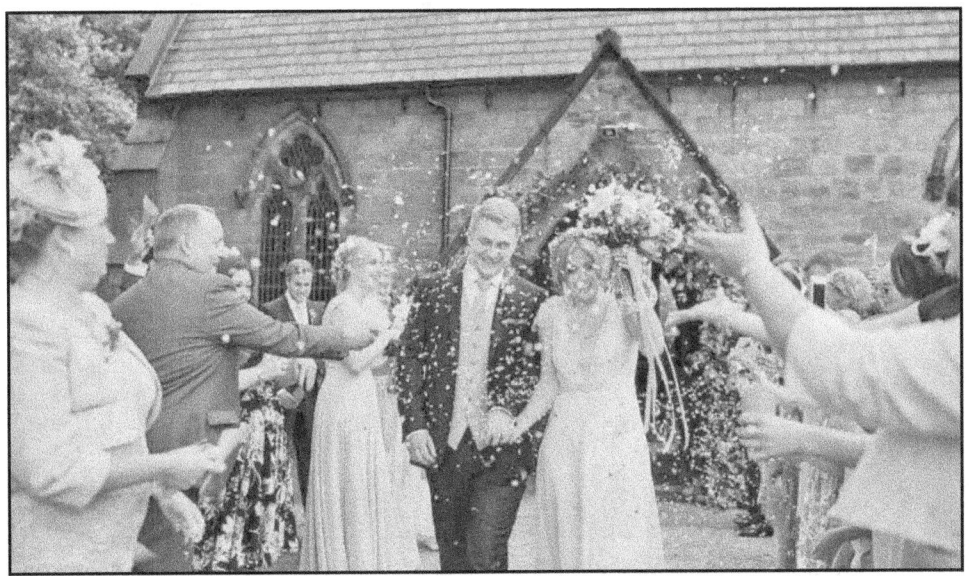

Another aspect of Events is our past. We may have had bad experiences in childhood. Or, as adults, we may have been involved in stressful situations, such as an accident, violence and so on. The issues arising from such events will usually have both short and long term effects.

HOUSING

Having a secure place to live is a major human need, and problems associated with that may trigger stress. Aside from the issue of homelessness itself, we come back to financial worries about being able to pay our rent or mortgage. But it may also be the case that our house needs some repairs, a new boiler, a new roof, it can seem endless. Moving house always rates highly on the stress tables, being a potent cocktail of financial pressures, dealing with legal issues, combined with relationship and perhaps work factors too

TIME CONSTRAINTS

A very common cause of immediate stress, given the pressures that many of us live under. We can become overwhelmed by the demands of family, work, and social schedules. Traditional work patterns are changing. People may be expected to work beyond their usual, set hours. Others work irregular hours (either because of shift work or zero hours type contracts), or fewer hours than they would like.

Both of these situations can create stress for workers. It makes childcare provision difficult (through cost or logistics). It may interfere with family or social activities, and so on. Children and teens are not exempt; they too have hectic schedules and an increasing pressure to succeed at extra-curricular activities. Add family commitments into the mix and we can see how

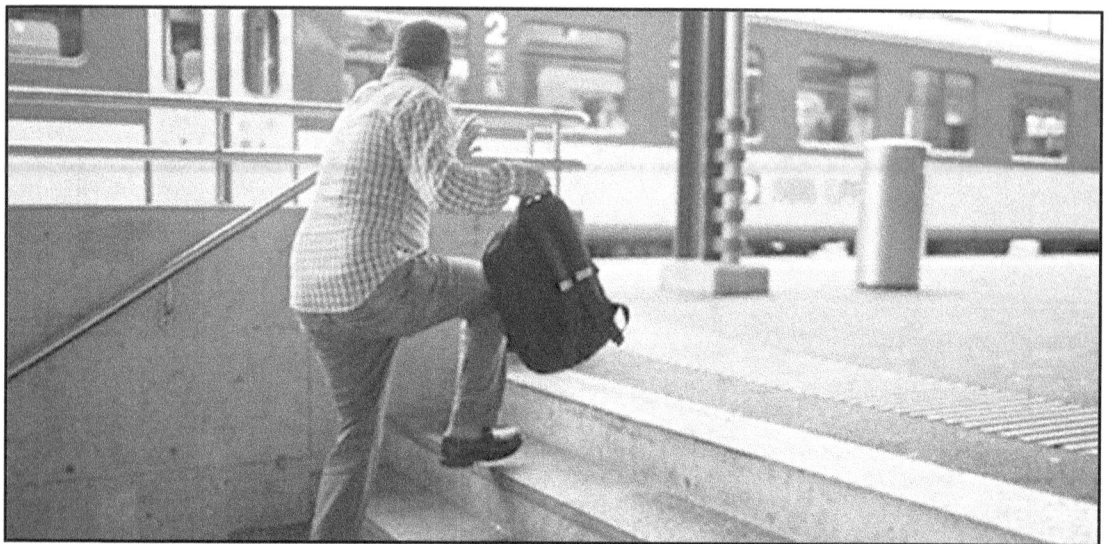

never enough hours in the day becomes the norm. We rush from one task to another, never quite finishing one. We may even feel guilty about taking some time out for ourselves, just sitting and doing nothing for a bit.

Lack of time may also have an effect on our sleep patterns - perhaps we stay up late at night to finish a report, or find ourselves getting up super-early to complete some task. We may also come to resent those who make demands on our time - an elderly relative, perhaps, even our own children at times. This can lead to guilt which, in turn, creates more stress.

Time stress can be insidious, in that it can actually be promoted as a "Good Thing!" I once worked in an office where to be at your desk after hours was to be seen as being keen and eager to "get on." It didn't matter what you were doing in that time (for me, I was killing time before going to my evening class once a week), just the fact that your were seen was enough to prove your commitment to the job.

Other places may promote that view even more vigorously, with staff strongly encouraged to work unpaid extra-hours, to come in early or stay late to "help out." It can be a slippery slope, leading to stress and burn-out (at which point you are replaced by someone "more keen.")

We see this culture heavily promoted in advertising and the media. The idea of the "go-getter" whose amazing lifestyle is filled to the brim with power lunches, a thrusting career and a full-on, hip social life. They never seem to to do laundry, take the dog for a walk or get a cold - because it is a fantasy! The problem is, these fantasies can become the basis for aspirations. People set unrealistic goals for themselves and fall into the trap of thinking "success" equals living a certain lifestyle. We don't have to be the perfect partner, the perfect parent, the best worker ever. At least, not at the expense of our own physical and mental well-being.

The converse can be having too much time on our hands. Perhaps through being retired, out of work, or being at home to look after the kids. We may feel our life lacks structure, that one day becomes just the same as another. In such case it can be easy to sink into lethargy, or even depression.

CHANGING CIRCUMSTANCES

Most of us settle into routines and get comfortable with them. When something comes along that disrupts that routine, it might trigger stress. It might be quite a minor thing, such as a change of shifts, it could be something major like a divorce! Change is not always negative, such as getting a promotion at work. But with that promotion comes extra responsibilities, new pressures. Maybe a child is leaving home, perhaps you are taking in a lodger?

WIDER ISSUES

So far, most of the Triggers we have discussed have been personal but we live and function in the wider word too. There may be less directly personal issues that trigger anxiety - politics, crime, the environment, the economic situation and so on. As I write this in the UK, we are still mired in the uncertainty of Brexit, which has been the most divisive political situation I have ever experienced (and I'm old enough to remember Mrs Thatcher and the Miners' strikes!) Such wider issues can have a deeper effect on us. We feel we have little or no influence over them, however, each may effect our lives quite considerably.

FEARS

The horror author HP Lovecraft famously wrote: *"The oldest and strongest emotion of mankind is fear, and the oldest and strongest kind of fear is fear of the unknown.*

That may well be true, there are universal unknowns that we all respond to - the big questions in life, for example.

Fear is a manifestation of stress and, similarly, may be positive as well as negative. A feeling of fear is a good thing if we are crossing a field that contains a bull, for example. That fear helps keep us aware and potentially assists should we need to make a quick run for it! That is presuming we do not let the fear take us over completely, something we shall be returning to later on.

There are other types of fears, such as phobias. These are more long term conditions and can range from the light (I don't like spiders!) to the serious (a person unable to leave their house because of agoraphobia). Other things, such as a fear of public speaking, may act as inhibitors to our social and professional lives.

KEEPING A JOURNAL

These are some possible Stress Triggers, then. Please don't read this as a list of things to get stressed about! The aim of the list is to help us start to recognise which events are responsible for the stress in our lives. There are two parts to this process - the first is to recognise that we are getting stressed.

You would be surprised by how stressed and tense people can become without them even realising it. This is because our stress has become normalised - what should actually be a short term condition has become our everyday mindset. The same goes for physical tension - people often don't realise how locked up their muscles are until you help shift them back into their natural movement patterns. Unchecked stress builds "armour" around the body. The odd thing is that it is not always there to keep bad things out, but most often to keep the stress locked in!

Once you get into the exercises later on, particularly the breath work, you will find it much easier to monitor your stress levels. You will have a baseline of comfort to work from, and will begin to learn which indicators to watch out for. As a start point, refer back to the section on Adrenal Dump. Heart rate, shallow breathing, the shakes, butterflies in the stomach, these are all very all clear indicators that the body is undergoing stress.

Once we know how to identify when we are stressed, we can begin to monitor it. A journal can be a great tool for doing this, as well as helping pinpoint those triggers. It doesn't have to be particularly complex or detailed, just keep a note of how you have felt on a particular day. For example:

Monday - 8.15am drove into work. Roadworks, heavy rain. Got agitated waiting in traffic queue.

It can be as simple as that. Where possible, try to add to your journal as soon as possible after the event. You don't even have to write it, you could record on your phone or similar. Perhaps someone has invented an App for this! Build a format for your reports. You might want to include:

Time and place
Particular conditions
Actions of others
How did that make me feel?
Stress scale of 1-5, where 1 is "peeved" and 5 is "bloody furious!"
Was the situation resolved?

Over even a short period of time, you will quickly build up a "stress picture." Looking back over it, you can hopefully begin to pick out patterns, those particular situations and issues that are most likely to act as triggers. You may also see how unresolved stress builds throughout the day, prompting a stronger reaction later on to even minor situations.

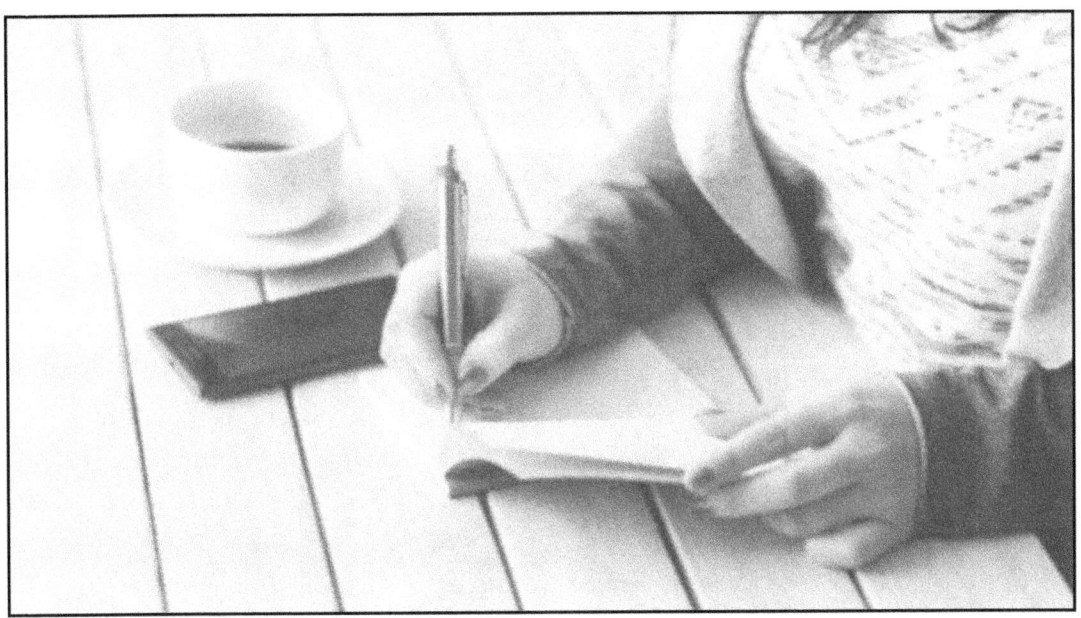

THE RUNNING COMMENTARY METHOD

This is actually a method of awareness training used by professionals in certain occupations, or by anyone wishing to increase their general overall observation and analysis skills. However, with a slight tweak, we can also use it as a Stress Monitoring tool.

The observation method is a simple idea. As we are driving, for example, we keep up a commentary of what we can see and what we are doing.

"Indicating, turning left into Fourth Avenue. Young man at kerb, wearing a jean jacket and black trousers, has a poodle on a lead."

That sort of thing. For our purposes, we point the commentary inward rather as well as outward.

"Turning left into Fourth Avenue. Man at kerb is stepping out - idiot! Can't you see I'm indicating, you moron! Hang on, getting annoyed, it's okay, calm down."

Obviously this is not always practical, though in some situations you can try maintaining an internal dialogue! This is a great way of monitoring stress "on the fly" and means, where possible, you can take instant action to reduce its effects.

Now we are able to identify stress, let's begin to look at some measures to manage its effects.

CHAPTER THREE
BREATHING

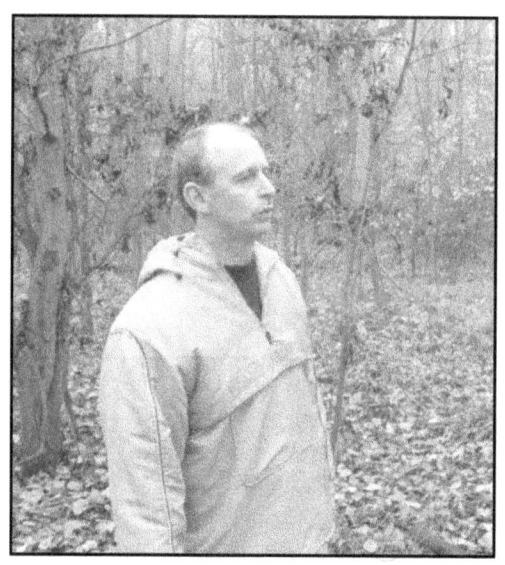

At the core of our stress management method is the simple action of breathing. Breathing is one of the few bodily processes that can either be voluntary or involuntary. It can take place automatically without thinking about it, or we can consciously alter it. The unique relationship between our thinking and our bodily processes, means that our breathing patterns play an important role in how we are affected by stress.

We breathe 24/7, sub-consciously most of the time, and that is where problems can begin. Over time, we lose track of our breathing, we lose sight of the connection between our mind and body. Have you ever wondered how a baby can scream so loudly for so long? Should you try and replicate this feat as an adult, I'm betting you will not only go hoarse quite quickly, you will also run out of puff within a few minutes.

The baby's secret is *belly breathing*. Babies usually indulge in diaphragmatic breathing, where the belly moves as the baby breathes in and out. We all are born with the ability to breathe in this way but tend to move on to chest breathing as adults, often to even more shallow breathing as we move into old age.

HOW BREATHING WORKS

The primary organs of the respiratory system are the lungs. Their function is to take in oxygen and expel carbon dioxide. Air, a mixture of oxygen and other gases, is inhaled. The nose and throat (trachea, or windpipe) filters the air. The trachea branches into two bronchi, tubes that lead to the lungs. The lungs add oxygen to the blood and remove carbon dioxide in a process called gas exchange. This exchange of oxygen and carbon dioxide takes place in the alveoli, small structures within the lungs. Once in the lungs, oxygen is moved into the bloodstream. Blood carries the oxygen through the body to where it is needed. Carbon dioxide in the blood is released back into the lungs, from where it is exhaled and the cycle begins again with the next breath.

During the process of inhalation, the lungs expand, a result of the contraction of the diaphragm and intercostal muscles (the muscles connected to the rib cage), thus expanding the thoracic cavity. Upon exhalation, the lungs recoil to force air out. The diaphragm is a dome-shaped muscle below the lungs that controls breathing. Usually, the diaphragm flattens out and pulls forward, drawing air into the lungs for inhalation. For exhalation the diaphragm expands up to force air out of the lungs. Adults normally take 12 to 20 breaths per minute. Strenuous exercise can drive the breath rate up to an average of 45 breaths per minute.

As well as a its physical effects, breathing also exercises a powerful influence on our psychological state. While this has been known and practiced for centuries in many traditions, modern science is just beginning to understand and corroborate the mind-breath-body

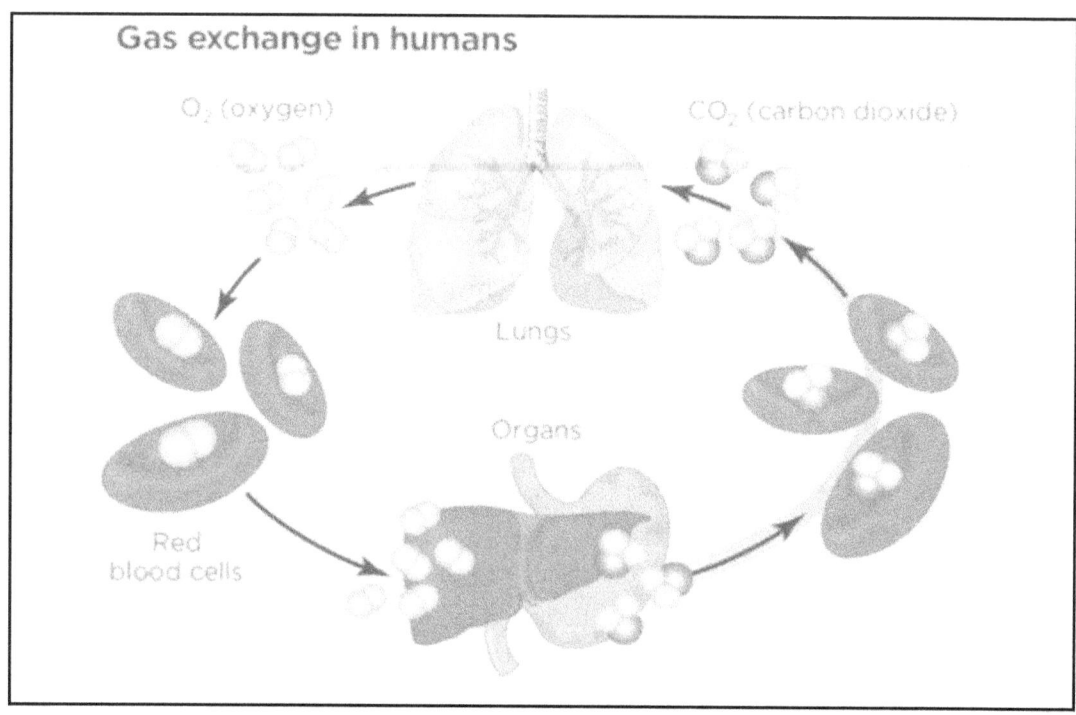

connection. As just one example, a recent study by researchers at Trinity College Dublin explained the neurophysiological link between breathing and attention. Their research showed for the first time, that breathing directly affects the levels of a natural chemical messenger in the brain called noradrenaline. This chemical messenger is released when we are challenged, curious, exercised, focused or emotionally aroused, and, if produced at the right levels, helps the brain develop new neural pathways. In other words, the way we breathe directly affects the chemistry of our brains in a way that can improve our brain health.

The study found that participants who focused well while undertaking a task that demanded a lot of attention had greater synchronisation between their breathing patterns and their attention, than those who had poor focus. The conclusion was that attention is influenced by our breath and that it rises and falls with the cycle of respiration. In this way, it is possible to optimise our attention by focusing on our breathing.

Other research has also shown that, there is evidence to support the view of a strong connection between breath-centred practices and a steadiness of mind. A study, conducted at North Shore University Hospital in Long Island, for example, showed that breathing manipulation activated different parts of the brain. These findings support the advice individuals have been giving for millennia: that during times of stress, focusing on one's breathing can actually change the brain. Exercises involving specific breathing patterns appear to alter the connectivity between parts of the brain and allow access to internal sites that normally are inaccessible to us.

BREATHING EXERCISES

Breathing, then, acts as a powerful link between our external and internal state. We can think of breathing as a bridge between the physical and the psychological. We already know that there is a link between the two, in any case. For example, if we have a physical ailment, say a toothache, that will impact us psychologically. We might get grumpy!

Likewise, psychological tension, such as stress or worry, will manifest in a physical way - hunched shoulders, scowling face.

The breath can act to connect the two and influence each directly and powerfully. Mentally focusing on the breathing will help the body to naturally relax. We can also consciously use it to get rid of tension. Likewise, doing forms of exercise or movement that involve coordinated breathing will help calm the mind, will bring us "into the moment."

One simple way we can practice conscious breathing, is through controlling the depth and length of our breath. As mentioned in the Introduction, this method is used in many traditions, from Taoist and Buddhist through to Orthodox Christian. Its use has become much more widespread in modern times, from athletic to military to health use. It even forms the base of the "burst breathing" methods used in

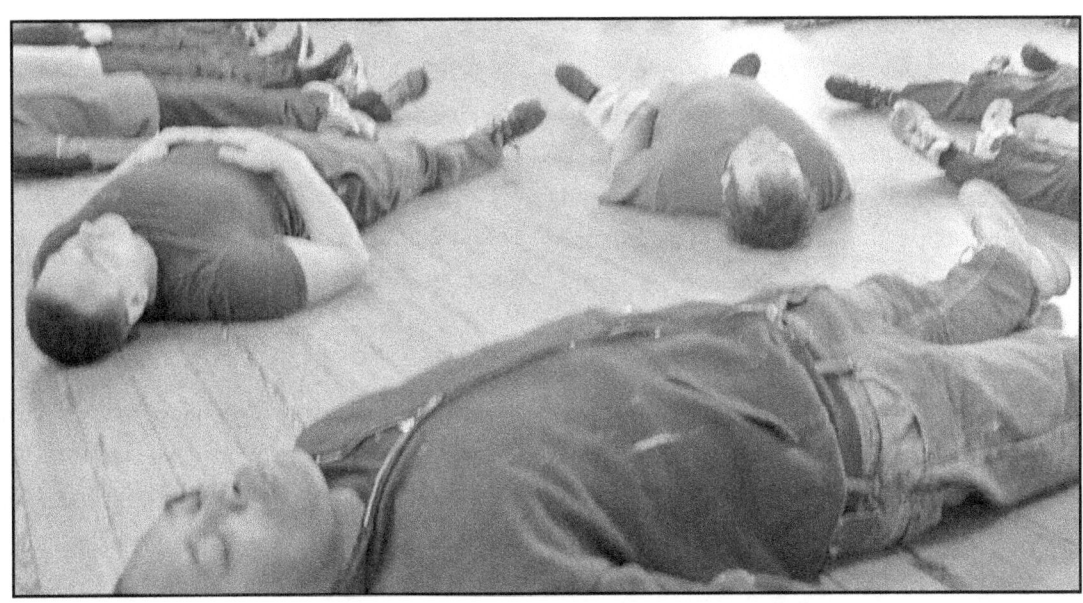

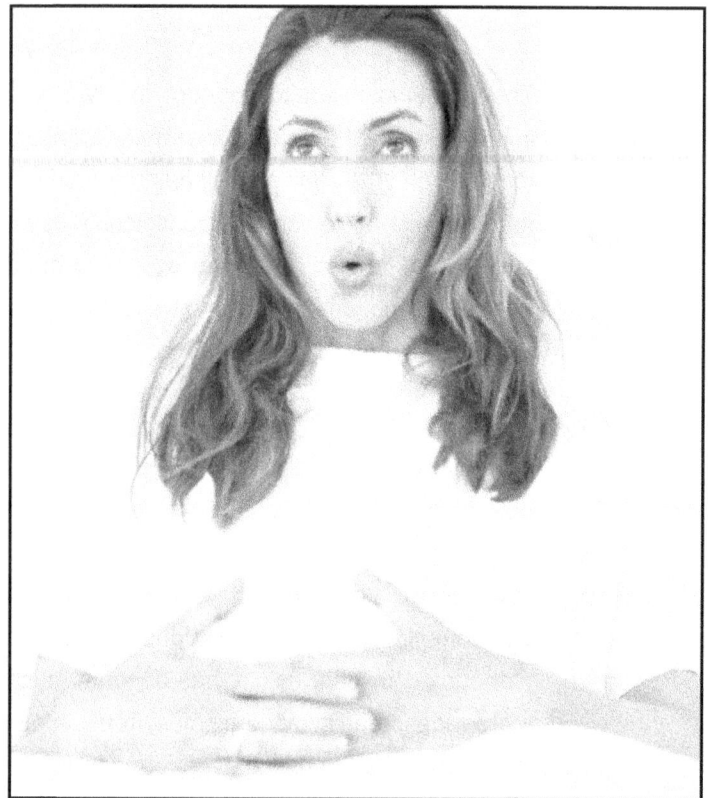
childbirth.

Breathing is about the only form of exercise I can think of where we can do no harm to ourselves. I cringe at some frantic fitness routines I see, that, when done with no thought of breathing or posture, can actually bring more tension into the body. With that comes a very real potential for short and long term damage. Breathing, however, can be practiced almost anywhere and by anyone. Having said that, there is one caveat - always be aware of your blood pressure, particularly when doing breath holds. If, at any time, you feel your blood pressure rising, come straight out the exercise, and do some Recovery Breathing is necessary (see later). If you do have blood pressure issues, always check with your Doctor before trying anything new. The practice of appropriate breathing exercises should help with many conditions but always work under medical advice.

We advise that you take your time with these exercises. Although we present them all here in one block, they should be practiced over a period of time, in a progressive way. Do not move on until you are comfortable with the previous method. Unless otherwise directed, all breathing for these exercises is *inhale nose, exhale mouth*. So, having established the two aspects to our breath work, depth and length, let's describe each, explain how they link together, then detail some basic breathing shapes. Later, we will add in our breath-work to movements and meditation-type practices.

DEPTH OF BREATHING

As we mentioned, when young we tend to breath "from the belly." Depth of breathing refers to how much of the lungs are used in the breathing. Breath drawn from the diaphragm will naturally involve more of the lungs than a shallow "in-out" breath. When done in a controlled way, each has its particular purpose.

Burst Breathing

The most shallow, this is also called Recovery Breath. The inhale is through the nose, then almost immediately out through the mouth. So the breath only just reaches the top part of the lungs, there is no expansion of the chest. Some liken this method to a dog panting, it certainly sounds similar!

Burst breathing is most often used to recover the breath if we are winded, or to help overcome immediate stress or duress. It is not done for very long, just long enough for us to recover or stabilise ourselves. It is a method commonly used during childbirth.

Chest Breathing

We can think of this as our everyday breathing, how we tend to be breathing when we are not thinking about it. The chest expands a little on the inhale and relaxes back on the exhale.

Deep Chest Breathing

This is how we breathe when we are consciously taking a deep breath, or yawning and stretching. The chest expands more to draw air deeper into the lungs. It's sometimes how people try and

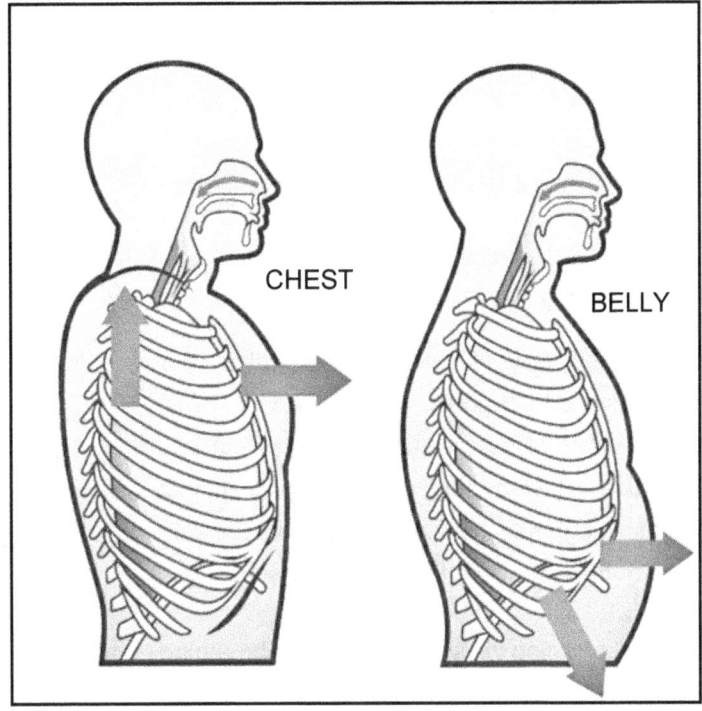

breath when they are out of breath (they would be better served by Burst Breathing.)

Belly Breathing

Also known as Diaphragmatic Breathing, the deepest of all. Air is drawn into the lungs by movement of the diaphragm. This is the method used by singers, martial artists and others. There are two versions, normal and reverse. For normal Belly Breathing, the diaphragm moves down, sucking air into the lungs. This pushes the belly out. On the out breath, the diaphragm relaxes, air passes out of the lungs and the belly flattens.

For reverse breathing, the diaphragm moves in and up on the inhale, pulling the belly in. On the exhale, the diaphragm pushes down to force the air out, and the belly expands.

With both methods, there is not so much obvious movement of the upper chest. However, the lower chest will be expanding, particularly around the back.

BREATHING SHAPES

One good way of learning to regulate our breathing is through the use of *shapes*. These are easy to remember and simple to put into practice. Having said that, things can get challenging when it comes to longer breaths and breath holds, so take things step by step.

When practicing the shapes, keep the breathing natural do not force anything. Maintain an even tempo throughout, do not speed up or slow down. Remember, if you experience any negative effects or feelings, come out of the drill and walk around for a bit.

CIRCLE BREATHING

Our foundation shape is the simple circle composed of two halves - an inhale and an exhale. Each half is of equal length. There will be a short, natural pause between each, but should be no breath holding at this stage. The breathing should be a gentle back and forth. Don't worry about length or depth of the breath to start with. At first it's simply enough to establish a conscious connection with your breathing. I always think that a room full of people practicing this sounds the sea coming in and going out on the shore, which is a nice image for the breathing itself.

TRIANGLE BREATHING

This adds in another "side" to the Circular Breathing in the form of a breath hold. The length of each remains equal. So the sequence is either inhale-hold-exhale or inhale-exhale-hold.

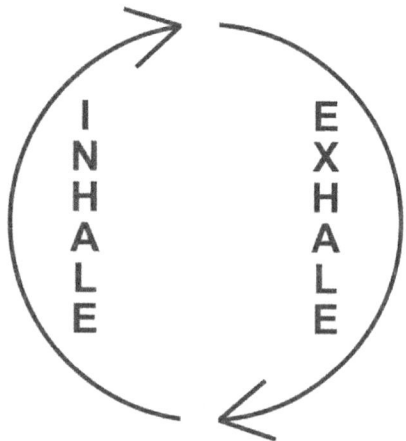
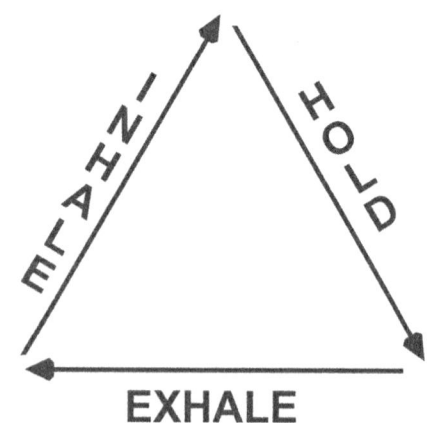

If you have not done any breath hold work before, then keep the sides quite short. The breathing needn't be too deep at this stage.

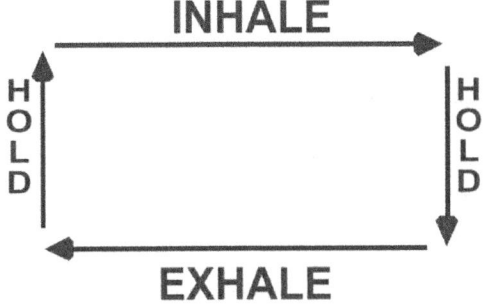

RECTANGLE BREATHING

Next we add in a second hold. So now the sequence is inhale-hold, exhale-hold. At first, we will keep the holds shorter than the breaths, in order to keep things comfortable.

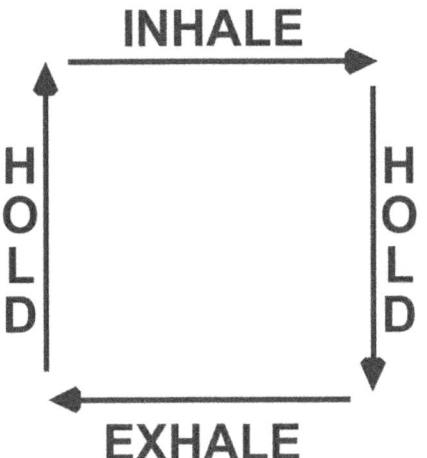

SQUARE BREATHING

Once you are used to holding the breath, the next progression is to make the holds equal length to the breathing. Remember to keep the whole sequence smooth and even. Imagine you are singing a note, it should be one clear tone, not a wavery or staccato sound! In fact, singers use very similar methods as part of their training.

Make sure when holding the breath that the body stays relaxed, particularly the chest area. Don't be tempted to try and take in a huge breath, keep everything natural as before.

How long the sides of each shape are are depends on the length of the breath. The easiest way to keep track of the length of breathing is by counting. So a four count square breath would go:

In - 2,3,4
Hold - 2,3,4
Out - 2,3,4
Hold - 2,3,4

These are our main breathing shapes. You should spend a little time practicing them, working through the progression from Circle to Square. Keep the length of each side comfortable to start. Length also depends on depth, it is best to stick to chest breathing to start and keep the count to around four or so.

LADDER BREATHING

The next thing to consider is improving control through extending the length of our breathing. This is where the ladder concept comes into play.

The basic idea of Ladder Breathing is to go into Circular Breathing with short breaths, and, step by step, increase the length of the breath. As mentioned before, we can count in our minds or use some activity, such as the number of steps while walking, as our measure. The main thing is to keep the counting consistent and always start low, build up, then go back down the ladder again.

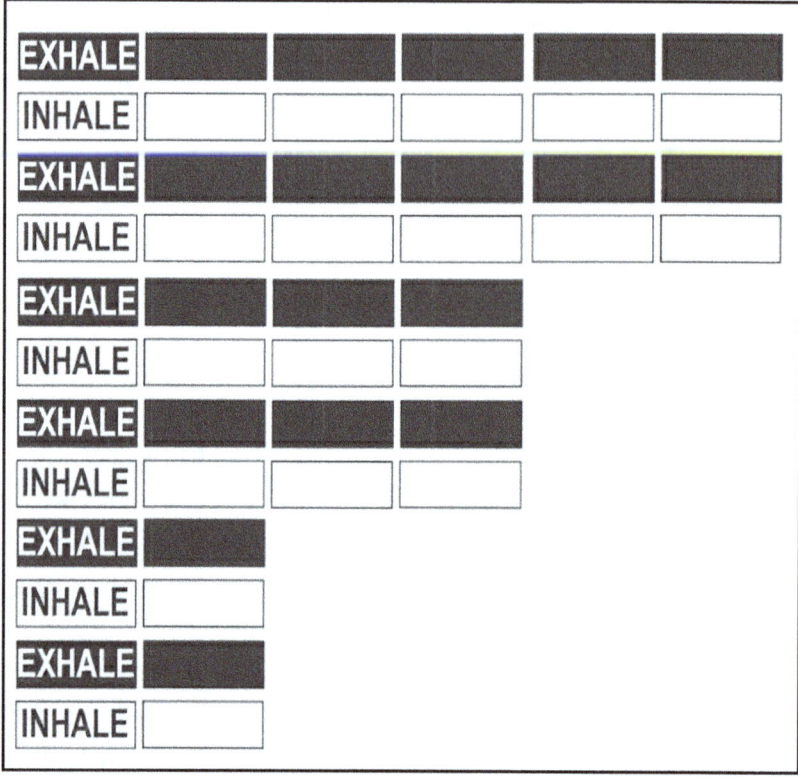

The diagram above shows how it works. The bottom rung of the ladder is a two count inhale, two count exhale. Then a four count, then a six count. The breath should be smooth across the count. So don't take a big gulp in on "one", spread the inhale across the count. At first, allow a short, natural pause between the inhale and exhale.

How long you spend on each rung depends on how much time you have. How high up the ladder you go depends on your breath control. As always, never force, build up slowly. You may find at the first your upper rung number is quite low but over time you will go up into double figures quite comfortably!

You can use whatever size "rungs" you want, I usually work in increments of in two. Once you reach your upper rung, you come back down in the same increments.

PYRAMID BREATHING

This combines the Ladder principle with any of the other shapes. You start with a short breath and gradually extend as you go up the ladder. Let's say we are using Square Breathing, so that's equal length breath and hold. The sequence will go:

Inhale for two
Hold for two
Exhale for two
Hold for two

Inhale for four
Hold for four
Exhale for four
Hold for four

Inhale for six
Hold for six
Exhale for six
Hold for six
And so on.

As with the Ladder, work up to your limit, then back down to two again. Spend as long as you like on each level. Later on, we will show you how to incorporate this method into activities such as walking and jogging, as well as describing its use in mindful movement.

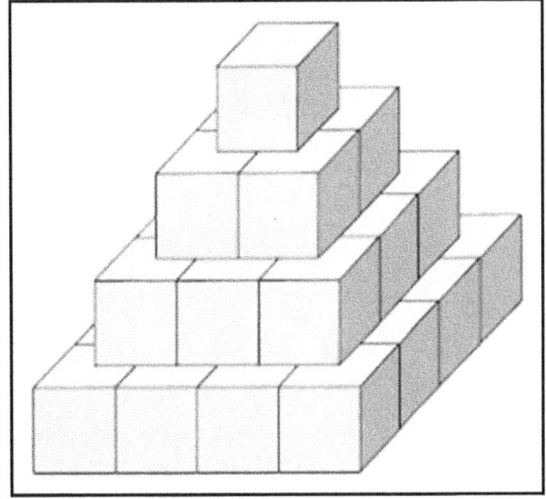

SHAPE AND DEPTH

There is an obvious correlation between length of breath and depth. Having said that, it is possible to burst breath using the diaphragm. In general though, the longer the breath the deeper it will be. When you do the Ladder Breathing, you will find the breath naturally getting deeper. You will also find, at some point, your natural "groove." This is the step where you have optimum breath length for whatever activity you are doing.

If you are jogging while practicing, once you have gone up and down the ladder, return to this step and stay on it. You should find it will really help with endurance - your body is working efficiently, you will also feel very focused.

CHAPTER FOUR
MANAGING EMOTIONAL TENSION

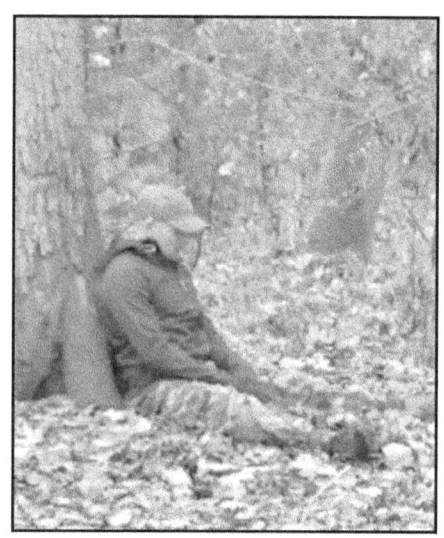

It would be fair to say that most of our everyday stress is in the mind. This goes back to our earlier comment about us living in the future or past - we worry about things that have happened, or things that may or may not happen in future.

We will first look at countering this by using methods to bring ourselves back to the here and now - methods that force the brain to think only of what is going on at the moment. We'll learn how to use breathing to calm the mind, to bring clarity and stillness to our racing thoughts.

Imagine you have a glass jar. You fill the bottom with dirt, then top it up with water. Put the lid on the jar and shake. The previously clear water will now be cloudy. If we set the jar down, the heavier dirt will gradually settle to the bottom and the water will become clear again. We are using the same principle with the mind. Our everyday brain is filled with swirling thoughts, they come and go in an endless procession, it can be hard to maintain any kind of focus. However if we sit quietly for a time and concentrate only on our breathing, those thoughts will slowly subside and we will be left with a wonderfully clear mind!

This simple practice can be surprisingly effective, you can come out of it feeling as though you just had a good sleep. This is because practicing these methods actually changes our brain states.

BRAIN STATES

Our brains have a unique set of waves. In neuroscience, there are five distinct brain wave frequencies, they are Beta, Alpha, Theta, Delta and Gamma. Each frequency, measured in cycles per second (Hz), has its own set of characteristics representing a specific level of brain activity and so a unique state of consciousness.

Beta (12-30Hz): normal waking consciousness, logic and critical reasoning. As we go about our daily activities we are in Beta state. Although important for everyday functions, higher Beta levels translate into anxiety. Some liken it to our *inner voice*, constantly chattering away.

Alpha (7.5-12Hz): the brain under relaxation, usually with the eyes closed, or while daydreaming. The relaxed, detached awareness achieved during light meditation is characteristic of Alpha state, which heightens imagination, memory, learning and concentration. Some describe Alpha state as the gateway to the subconscious mind, and call it *the voice of intuition.*

Theta (4-7.5Hz): the state of deep meditation and light sleep, including the REM dream state. Theta is the realm of the subconscious mind, normally only momentarily experienced as we drift off to sleep and arise from deep sleep. A sense of deep connection can be experienced at Theta, leading to inspiration and insight.

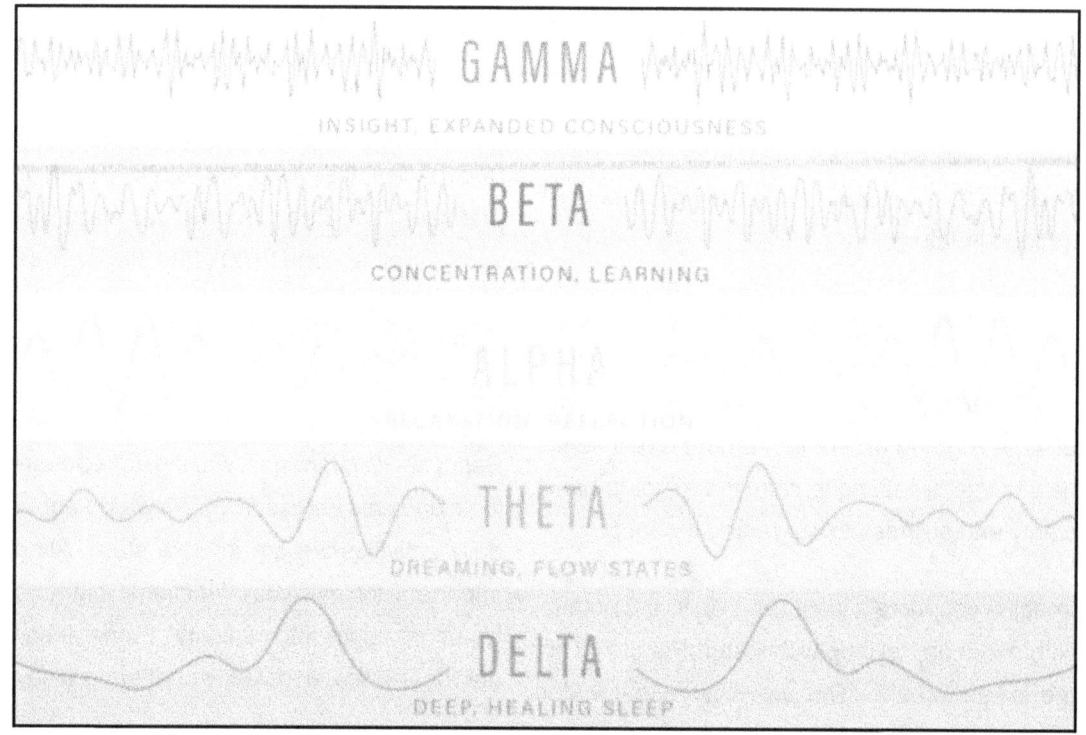

Delta (0.5-4Hz): the slowest frequency, present in deep, dreamless sleep and in very deep meditation, where awareness is completely detached. Delta is the realm of the unconscious mind and is associated with deep healing and regeneration, underlining the importance of deep sleep to our healing process.

Gamma (30-100Hz): the most recently discovered range, and the fastest in frequency. Little is known about this state of mind but initial research shows that Gamma waves are associated with bursts of insight and high-level information processing.

So let's first look at how we can use breathing methods to alter our brain state.

QUIET SITTING

The easiest method to calm our minds, Quiet Sitting can be done whenever you need to take a short break from things. You only need a few minutes to do it.

Sit quietly, close your eyes and begin Circle Breathing. Inhale nose, exhale mouth. Not too deep, remember, keep everything comfortable.

Maintain good posture, don't slump. Don't worry about counting the breath, just let it come and go.

Keep the mind focused on the breathing as much as you can and let all the muscles relax. You may find that thoughts spring up - don't fight them, just let them come and go. Don't analyse them or get sidetracked by them. If you find yourself drifting mentally, come back to the breathing. Inhale, exhale.

When you are done, slowly open the eyes and bring yourself back into the world. You may wish to stretch or move around a little before resuming your activities.

DEEP BREATHING

If we need to work deeper, we can use Diaphragm Breathing to really slow down both mind and body. This is a longer exercise than the Quiet Sitting, so you will need to set aside a more time. You may also want to change your environment to suit - dim the lights and so on.

Lie on your back on a flat surface with your knees bent. Place a pillow under your head your knees for support. Place one hand on your upper chest and the other on your belly, just below your rib cage and above your navel.

Now breathe in slowly through your nose, letting the air in deeply, towards your lower belly. The air going into your nose should move downward so that you feel your stomach rise with your other hand. The movement and airflow should be smooth, you shouldn't feel like you're forcing your lower belly out. The hand on your chest remains still, while the one on your belly rises up.

Next, let your belly relax. You should feel the hand that's over it fall inward. Again. don't force your stomach by clenching. Exhale through the mouth. The hand on your belly should move down to its original position.

At first, just practice this method for a few of minutes at a time. The diaphragm is like a big muscle, if we over-use it it will become a little sore and tender. As the diaphragm strengthens, you can gradually extend the length of the practice.

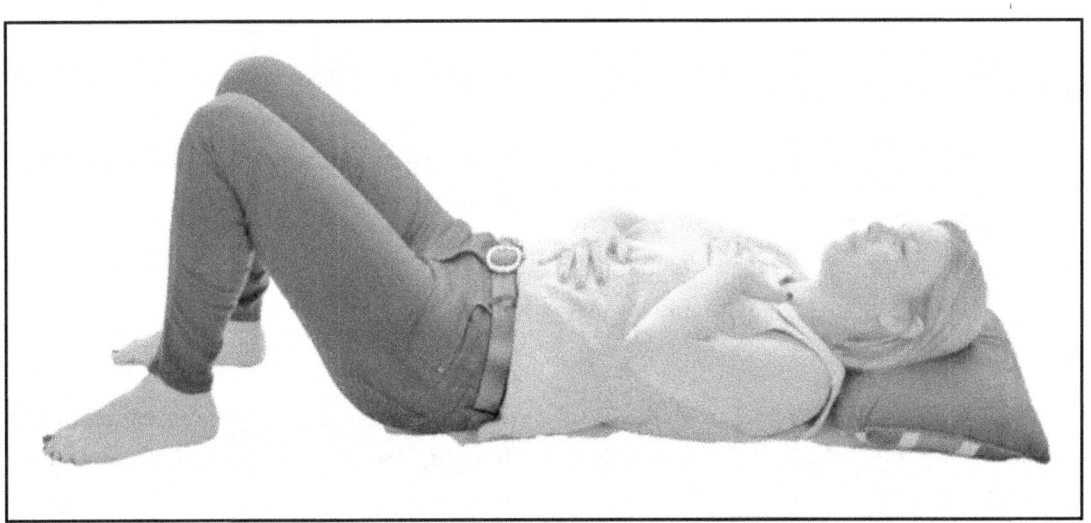

After practicing regular breathing from the diaphragm for a while, you might like to try Reverse Breathing. It gives a slightly different feel and, for me, allows even more air to be drawn into the lungs. Start from the same position. This time, on the inhale, draw the abdomen in and up, pulling the air into the nose. Again, the hand on the chest should not move very much. For the exhale, push down and out, squeezing the air out as the belly expands.

In both cases, keep the mind focused entirely on the breathing and the physical sensations - the rise and fall of your hands, the movement of the belly. Let all the other muscles relax, imagine you are sinking down into the surface beneath you. The breathing should naturally lengthen as you go on. Do not be tempted to rush straight into super-deep breaths, let them lengthen naturally.

When you are ready, slowly come out of the state by shortening the breaths a little and bringing the breathing back up into the chest. Think of it in the same way as you fall asleep and wake up, usually gradually. In fact, it is not uncommon for people to fall asleep while doing this exercise, which is why we advise you leave plenty of time to do it! As such, it's also a good method to use if you are having trouble sleeping at night.

Once done, get up slowly and stretch / move around a little before returning to your regular activities.

THOUGHT CONTROL

One of the biggest challenges in Quiet Sitting, or any mindful exercise, is what to do about thoughts. Whenever we sit still for more than five seconds, thoughts pop up unbidden and, before you know it, they are racing through the mind. One thought leads to another, there is no control over the direction they take. Eastern traditions call this *monkey mind*. The brain leaps to and for, from past to present to future, with no apparent aim or direction.

But what are thoughts? Thoughts are simply mental events and are usually a way of dealing with feelings. Think about how we develop as humans. A baby has little more than sensations and feelings. Thinking develops from learning to express those feelings and experiences.

Thoughts are an internalisation of our experience of the world; what Freud called the *reality principle*. All thoughts, as distinct from feelings, have a format derived from sensory images. So when we are feeling our way through a problem using thoughts, we are, as it were, feeling our way through a virtual form of reality, feeling our way through a representation of reality.

We could say that thinking creates a virtual space where we can work out, in the safety of our minds, what to do in relation to reality, before we actually put a solution into effect. In short, thoughts are the bridge between feelings and actions.

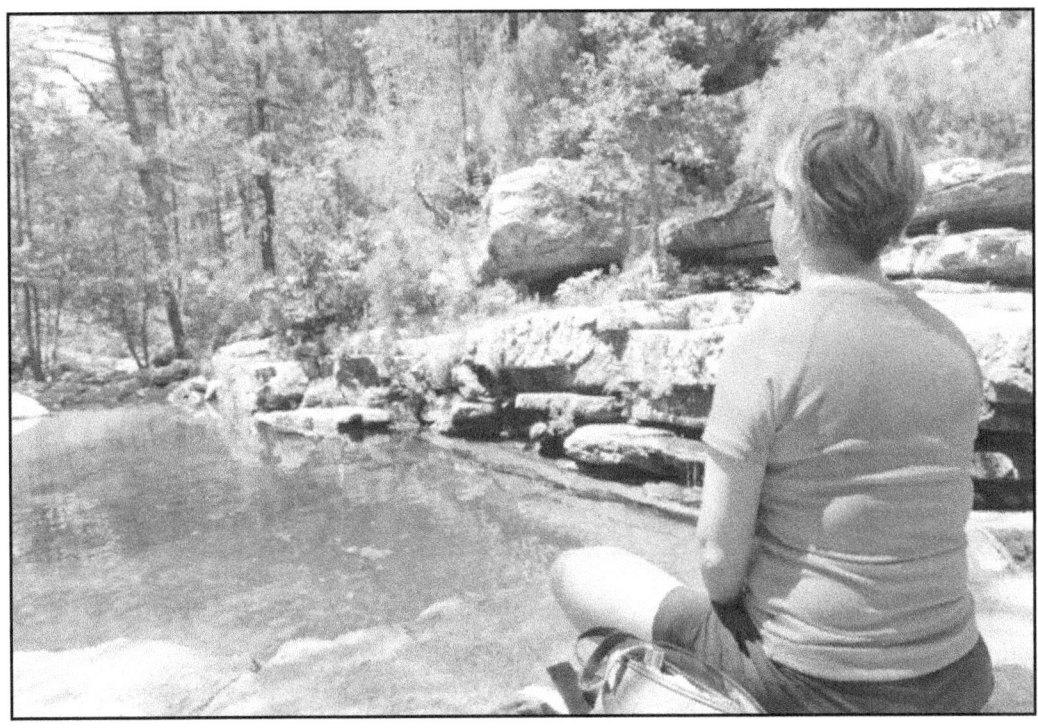

Thoughts can become very elaborate. We have a feeling that creates a thought, we can then think about that thought! Later on, we can even re-create that feeling via a particular thought. So once we understand our feelings, we should find that we have a lot more control over our thoughts. Were you ever scared of the dark as a child? The darkness creates a feeling of fear. The fear creates thoughts of what might be in the lurking in the dark - a monster, perhaps?

This, in turn, feeds the fear and drives us to the action of pulling the blanket over our head. Later on, we understand that there is no monster in the dark, so the fear generated thought does not arise. Or we may use a thought of something pleasant in order to counter the fear.

Much like breathing, then, thoughts and emotions are a two-way street. We can think ourselves miserable, and misery can overcome our rational thought. This does mean that we can use on to influence the other and gives us some ideas on how to deal with thoughts during meditation and similar practices.

The worse thing you can do is to try and stop your thoughts altogether, or try to fight them. Struggle will bring more thought and tension. Instead, we aim to either focus thoughts or to let them "run free."

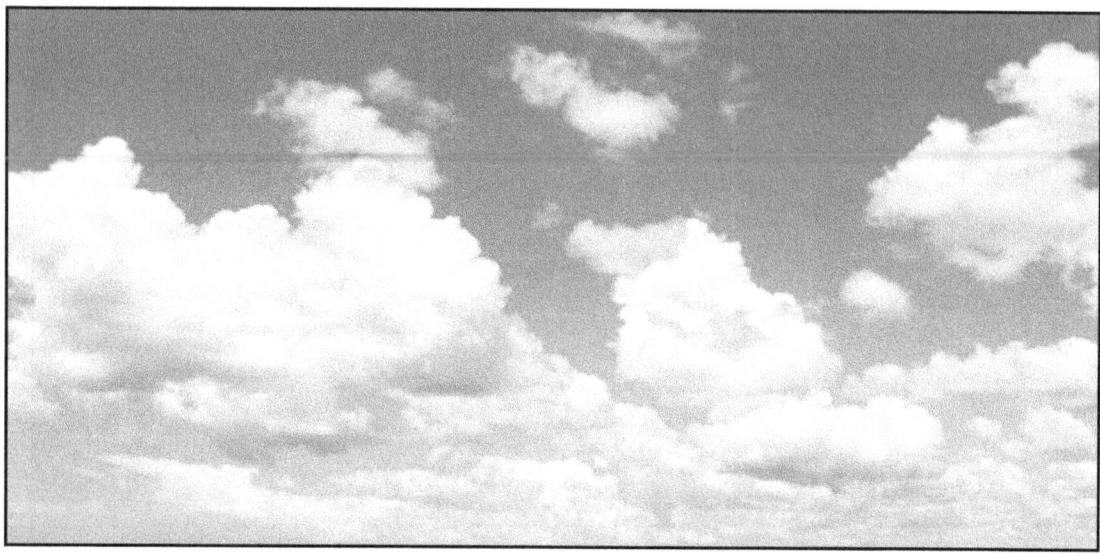

FOCUSED THOUGHT

Probably the most common way of controlling our thoughts at the start is by counting. Counting the breath serves a double purpose and helps keep the mind "on point." If the count wavers, go back to one and start over. You can work in cycles of ten to start with, count one to ten, then back to one.

Another method is to focus your thoughts totally on one single thing. Picture a rose in your mind. Imagine the rose turning, so that you see it from all angles. Note the colours, the texture of the petal, the stem. What is the scent of the rose? How does it feel if you brush your fingers against the petals?

In short, utilise all the senses but keep the focus narrow. If you find your thoughts straying at all, pull them back to the rose.

Something else you can try is to focus on a body part. Many Eastern traditions have you focus on the *dan tiens*, or *chakras*, what are termed *energy centres* of the body. This focus may be accompanied by physical sensations and tied in with specific breathing patterns. You don't have to be knowledgeable about these points, you could focus on the sensation in your hands, for example.

The final option we will discuss is the method of using sound. We use a repetitive phrase over and over, either out loud or in the mind. We use this phrase to keep the mind focused, to keep any other thoughts suppressed.

What phrase you use is up to you. Eastern traditions may use a mantra, such as the Buddhist *om mani padme hum*. Other traditions use prayer, such as the Orthodox Christian

Jesus Prayer, *Lord Jesus Christ, have mercy on me, a sinner.* Any suitable phrase will do. By suitable I mean something that is personal to you and is positive. In fact, you can use a positive phrase to help boost the benefits of the exercise, what is known as affirmation.

LETTING THOUGHTS GO

An alternative option is to exercise no control over our thoughts at all. We simply let them arise as they may. Think of the thought as a cloud - you watch it as it sails gently past but don't get attached to it. You may notice that the thought causes an emotion or sensation to arise in the body. That's okay, just observe that, too, then bring your focus back to the mind. With practice, you will find that random thoughts pop up less frequently. We are back to that notion of the muddy water in the jar gradually becoming clear again.

A side effect of learning to deal with our thoughts in our quiet work is that we can apply exactly the same methods to thoughts that arise during the day, or in stressful situations. It doesn't matter if it is a fear-based thought or an angry or aggressive one, we can use the above methods to counter it.

Don't attach to it, let it go, don't act on it. We've all heard the old adage *take a deep breath and count to ten*, right? Or the more modern version - *never send the first e-mail!*

MINDFULNESS

Mindfulness means being aware of our inner and outer state, and may be added in to any type of movement. This is very good from a stress management perspective as it focuses our attention entirely on the movement and moment at hand. We are engaged fully in the present, rather than worrying about the future or the past. This gives our brains a rest from our worries, can alleviate the physical symptoms of anxiety and also help us discover a simple joy in our movements and physicality.

Disciplines such as Tai Chi, martial arts, yoga, etc are all examples of Mindful Movement. They

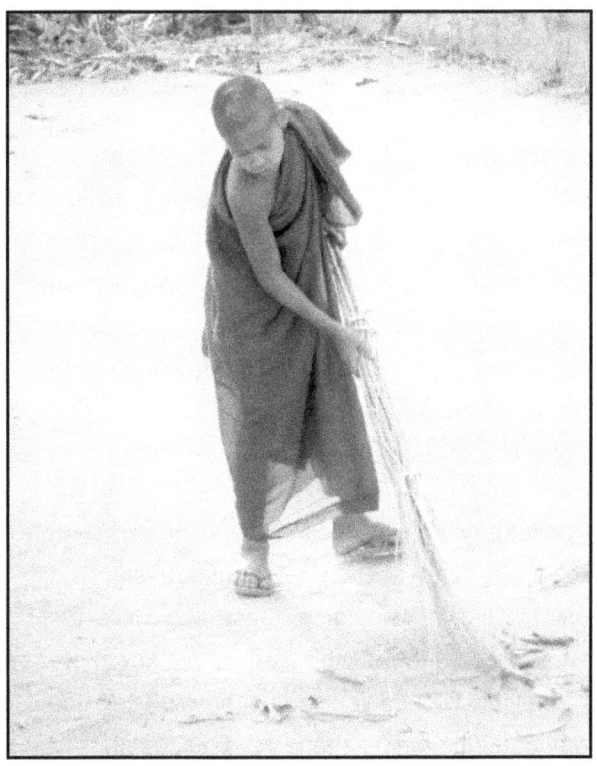

can be very detailed, though, and take a lot of time to learn. If you want to try something more straightforward, or if you want to experiment with putting mindfulness into your every day activities, try this.

The next time you have to do something, put an awareness of your breathing and posture into it. Let's say you have to sweep up the leaves in the yard. Normally, you might put in some earbuds and listen to some music while you do this mundane task. Instead, before you begin, hold the broom and go into Circular Breathing. Be aware of your body, your posture. Are you carrying any undue tension? Be aware of physical sensations - is there a cold wind blowing on your face?

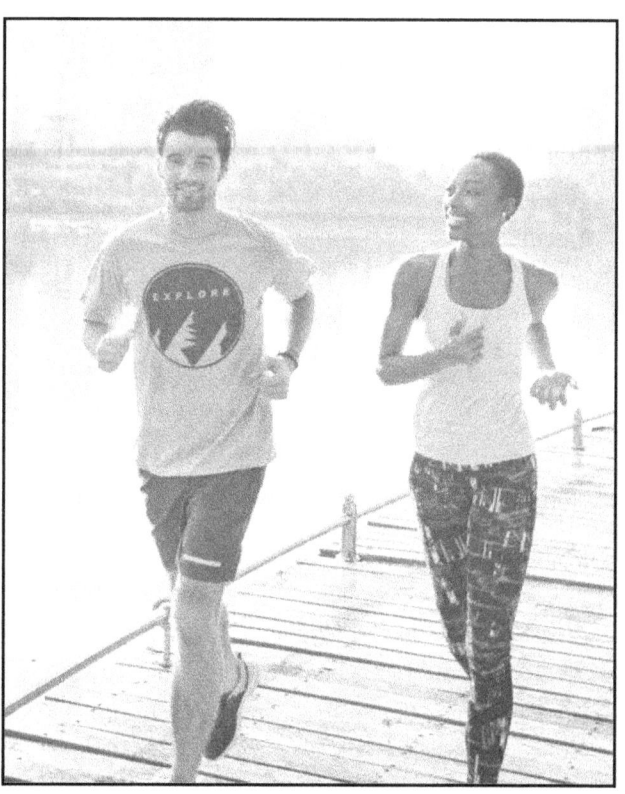

Continue breathing and next *listen*. What can you hear? The hum of passing traffic? Bird-song? Spend a couple of minutes in this state before you being sweeping. Now, as you sweep, inhale as you lift the broom, exhale on the sweep. Build into a rhythm, following your breath. Relax your shoulders. Look around, you are a part of your environment.

Think about nothing but the task in hand. When the job is done, spend another minute standing still in Circular Breathing. Once you have the idea, it is easy to work this method into any chore - particularly ones you find boring! You can use any of the breathing shapes as you see fit.

LADDER WALKING & RUNNING

Walking is another every day activity that we can practice mindfullly. It's also a great form of exercise. This time, we will work with Ladder Breathing, keeping count by the number of steps we take. So begin build inhaling for two steps, exhaling for two and climb through the sequence from there. Remember, once at the top, you come back down again.

The length you stay on each step depends how long your walk is. Even with a short walk you should be able to get up to eight and back down again. Make sure you maintain a constant speed

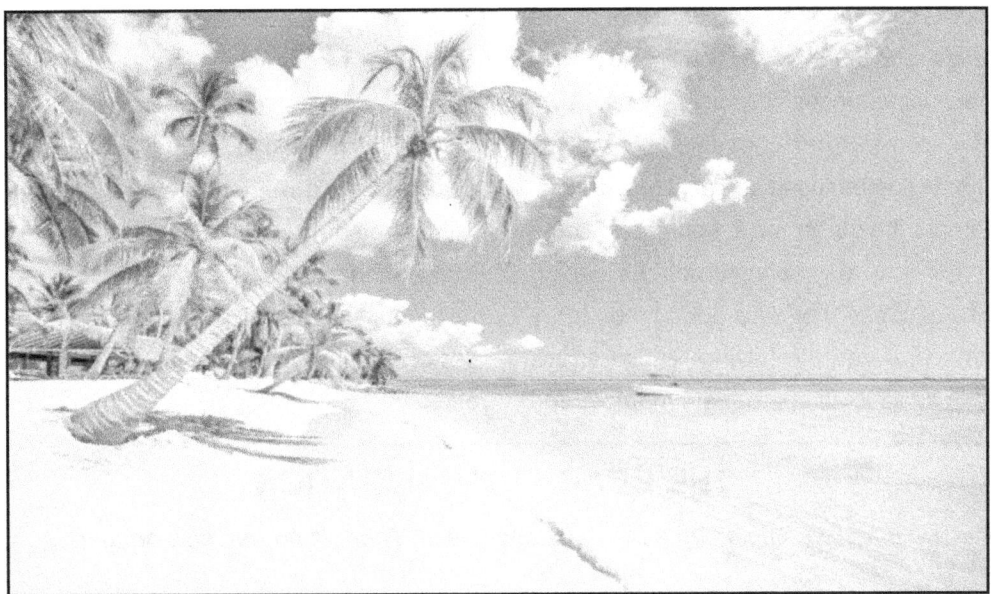

- as the breaths become longer it can be tempting to speed up the walk a bit!

One other piece of advice - keep your mobile phone in your pocket, or even at home! As you walk, look about you, take in your surroundings! This is the first step to linking our inside state with the outside world. You can do the same method if your are out jogging. I use it when taking the dogs for a run.

VISUALISATION

Our next exercise takes the concept of Quiet Sitting and adds in another layer - *visualisation*. Now, rather than just focusing on our breathing or a physical sensation, we use our imagination to create a vision. We touched on this with the rose earlier but this is a more involved version of that method.

We typically do this in order to remove ourselves mentally from a situation. That may be something that is happening to us right now. For example, the last time I used it was when sat in the dentist chair for root canal treatment! It may be used to get a bit of time "away from it all." In a sense, you can think of it as a waking dream, or a day dream, but a focused one, rather than just drifting away.

In addition, we can use a visualisation to create a *Happy Place*. In essence, this is a calm space, a mental construct that we can retreat to in times of stress. While it can take a little time to build up a visualisation, we can use a method called *anchoring* that will immediately take us to our place. So there are three steps to this process: build the visualisation, create the Happy Place, create an anchor to that place.

A visualisation can be used in isolation, of course, depending on how much time we have and the circumstances. It is not something we should use when our complete attention is required on something - such as when driving, for example. If you are on a boring train ride, though, or you are having trouble sleeping because of stress, both are good times to try this method. If you are having regular stress episodes and it is an appropriate method, add in the Happy Place and anchor in order to allow yourself to access your visualisation quickly. We give you an example visualisation below, and you can download an audio version of this using the links given in the Appendices.

It is also good to develop your own visualisations, based on pleasant memories and good experiences. These will be much stronger as they will be uniquely personal to you.

THE BEACH VISUALISATION

Picture yourself walking along a lovely, sunny beach. There is no-one else around.

Hear the gentle hiss of the waves on the sand as you inhale and exhale.

Your feet sink into the warm sand. Wiggle your toes. Feel the warmth of the sun on your skin. Let your muscles relax.

A cool, refreshing breeze ruffles your hair. You hear the distant gulls. You smell the salt air, and suntan lotion.

Ahead, is a sun lounger. You sit in it and recline into the soft padding. Paint the scene in your mind, make the colours bright and vivid, the sensations real and pleasant.

Relax and sink back into the comfortable lounger as the waves and your breathing become slower.

Feel the energy of the sea. Feel how you connect to that energy. Your breath is the wind and waves.

Each time you exhale, let go of something you don't need. Worries, stress, tension, all flow away into the sea

Stand and keep looking at the beach.

To finish, slowly open your eyes and come back to the here and now.

Step one, then, is to create our vision. The physical requirements are the same as our earlier breathing exercises, seated or laying down in a comfortable position. Close your eyes, begin Circular Breathing and let mind and body settle down. Once everything is calm, we switch on our imagination and go into our visualisation.

THE ANCHOR

Once able to visualise a scene, we can make it a Happy Place that you can repeatedly visit. To do this this, run through the same procedure as above but add this section in just before finishing:

Look around at the beach again. This place is always here for you. It is yours and yours alone. It is safe and warm here. You can return at any time, this place is always here waiting for you.

We now add in our anchor. This is an impulse stimulus or trigger which causes a specific response, which is always the same. In contrast to a reflex, this response is learned and not hereditary. The basic principle was discovered by the Russian scientist Pavlov during his famous experiments with dogs.

Anchors can occur in all sensory systems. The word *visualisation* implies sight, but you might like to experiment with the use of scents and smells as triggers as well as . Smell has a very direct connection to memory, a certain scent can transport us instantly back to a very specific place and time.

For the purpose of this exercise, we will choose a physical anchor, something very simple but definite. Once immersed in our scene, we will make a fist with one hand, but tucking the thumb inside the fist rather than outside. Now squeeze the fingers, putting pressure on the thumb. Do this a few times, with each squeeze the scene becomes more and more vivid in your mind.

The anchor can be any movement or action similar to the above. It is best to choose something that is not an everyday movement, something a little unusual. With a little practice you will find you can trigger your vision quite easily.

Your visualisation can be of anything, it doesn't even have to be a real experience. You might imagine singing on stage with your favourite group, or flying high through the clouds on the back of a dragon! The key is to make your initial visualisation as vivid and real and possible in your mind. Involve all the senses, really put yourself into the experience.

It might sound strange, but this is a surprisingly effective method. Our imaginations are much more powerful than we think and, as we have already established, what goes in our mind has a profound effect on our body. Boring or unpleasant situations may never be the same again!

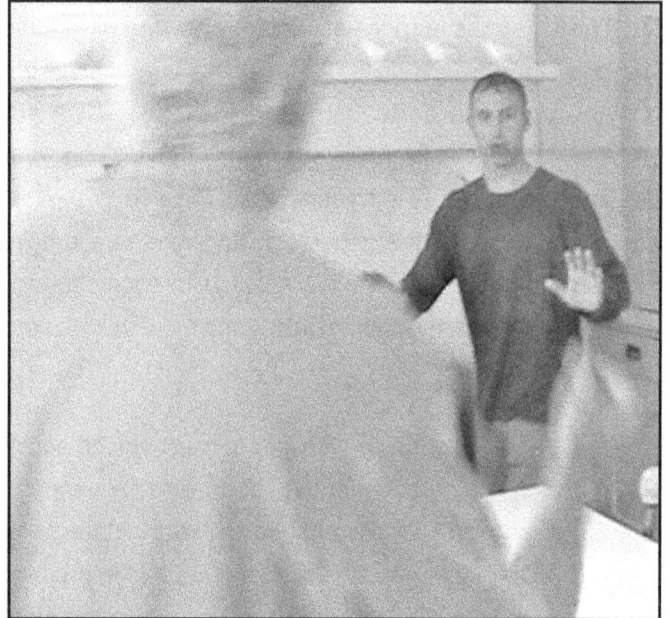

GENERAL MINDSET

Our first stress management methods have been techniques to help calm the mind post-stress. Let's now think of some ways we can prevent stress from getting a grip on us in the first place. One thing to consider is our mindset in general. We will start by thinking about *perspective*.

PERSPECTIVE

What this means is understanding the relative scale of a situation, placing any resulting stress in its proper context and maintaining a sense of perspective about the whole experience. Sometimes a minor event can trigger a major stress response, showing, perhaps, that there are unresolved underlying issues of tensions present. Framing everything in its proper place can help us prioritise the issues we need to deal with, and also highlight how stress can build over time until we are tipped "over the edge."

If we are using our journals regularly we begin to identify our major Stress Triggers. Let's take one as an example to illustrate how we can then work to frame it.

"I bumped into someone on the way into work, he turned and swore at me. I immediately got angry and felt very aggressive towards him. Luckily he stormed off before I could respond."

The first step is to understand the context of the situation and our own role in it. In this case, I bumped into the other guy, so the situation was of my own making. Perhaps I then didn't apologise, making the other person even more angry. From his viewpoint, a guy has barged into him, then not said sorry. He has every right to feel angry!

Switching viewpoints is another powerful method for gaining perspective on a situation. This means not only seeing things from the others person's point of view, as above, but also understanding that person's circumstances and experiences. We might imagine, for example, that the person in the scenario above is having a bad day. Late for work, facing threat of redundancy, just heard that his mother has to go into hospital. Our intrusion into his life suddenly gives him a focus for all that anger and frustration. With that in mind, we could modulate our response accordingly and hopefully defuse the situation before it goes any further.

The same thing applies back onto us - is this other person actually nothing more than a handy target for me to vent all my stresses on? Do they deserve to bear the brunt of all my problems? In terms of perspective we should then work to frame this incident in the wider scheme of things. A brief incident in a busy day in a city full of millions people rushing to work, in a world full of people, most of them struggling just to survive, In the broader context, it seems silly to get stressed and argumentative over such a minor thing. It is often our ego that gets pricked and rears up in confrontation, and for what? Put it in context, apologise, breathe, move on.

One thing that may help with the sense of perspective is to think of the future. Tomorrow, next week, a month's time, this incident will be nothing more than a dim memory, if handled correctly. If handled incorrectly, you might get into a fight and end up in court! Future outcomes can be difficult to plot but one thing is clear - no-one ever got into trouble through walking away from a pointless argument.

Framing things in time may also help with more serious issues. Sometimes we can see no end to a problem. It may be difficult, but perhaps we have to have a little faith that things will improve. It might be in a relationship context, it may be financial. That doesn't mean doing nothing and relying on wishful thinking. It does mean keeping a positive mindset and taking what steps we can to improve the situation.

ACCEPTANCE & DENIAL

That brings us on to our next issue. I'm sure you will have the Serenity Prayer before:

God, grant me the serenity to accept the things I cannot change,
  Courage to change the things I can,
    And wisdom to know the difference.

This simply means that if we are unable to directly influence a situation, we should not unduly worry about it. If we are able to directly influence a situation, then we should take the steps to do so. In order to achieve this, we have

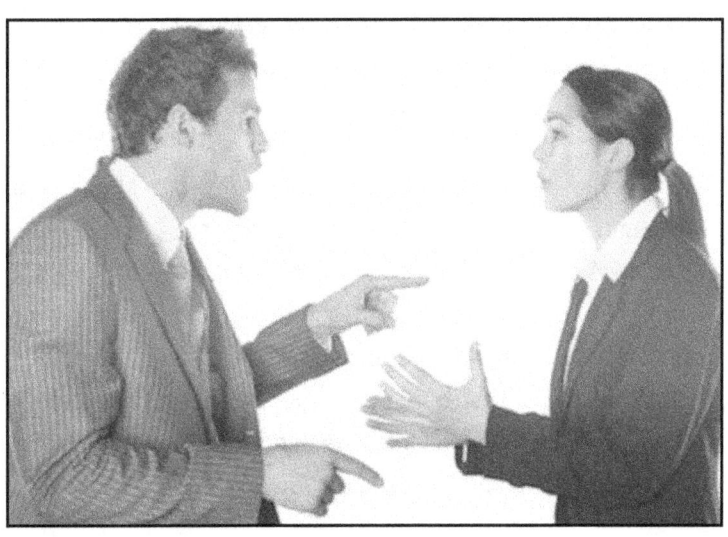

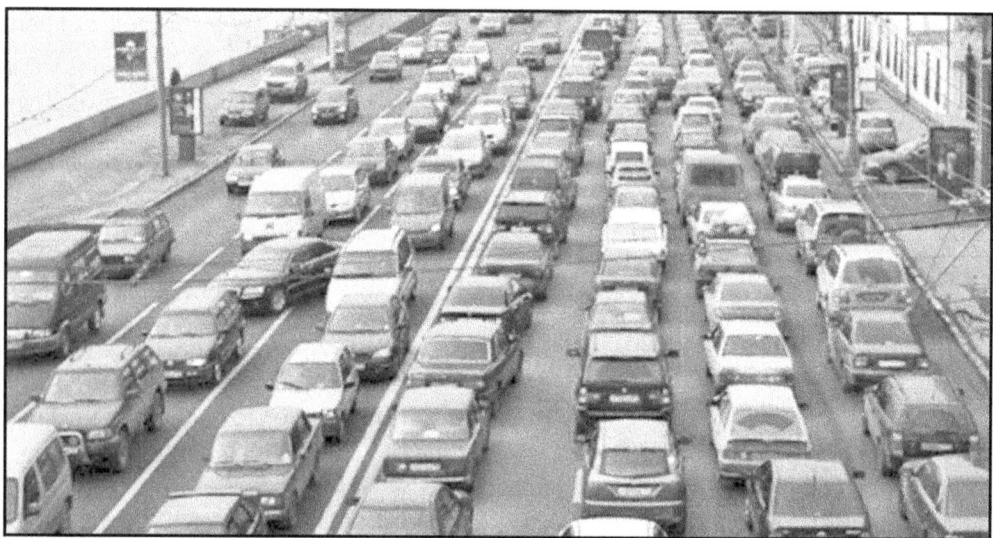

to understand *acceptance*.

There's a brutal truth about life that we all have to learn to accept - we have no control over many of the things that happen to us. In fact, when we really come down to it, there is very little we have control over at all, not even ourselves at times! If we start at the level of inter-personal relationships, people can be stubborn, unpredictable (in good and bad ways) and not always receptive to our, no doubt, excellent advice and suggestions!

Wider issues in our daily life are usually beyond our control - traffic, the weather, how things are structured at work. If we look beyond that, we have to live in and deal with economic and political issues, environmental and ecological concerns, civil unrest, even war. Our first step, then, should be to recognise those things which are beyond our control, or, at least, beyond our immediate control if we are involved in a situation.

So, we have to accept those things we can not control. That doesn't mean we have to like them, nor does it mean we have to be totally submissive to everything that is happening to us. What it does mean is we have to learn to *let go* and not worry about those issues.

Denial can be a powerful force and one we use more often than we might think. Have you ever seen the reactions of people in a stressful or shocking situation? Observe how some cover their ears or eyes. It is as though they are trying to "shut out" the horrible thing they are witnessing, another aspect of our freeze response, perhaps. When people fall, they often stiffly put it their hands out in an attempt to stop the fall, to "deny" it, usually resulting in injury. A trained martial artist learns to accept the fall and smoothly rolls into it without harm. Mental acceptance tends to bring physical relaxation with it, again this is the aim of the martial arts. People used to movie fights are often surprised to learn that the higher level martial artists are all trying to become more relaxed, not tense. Part of that process is learning to accept what is happening to you and respond to it, rather than deny or resist the situation.

Denial tends to restrict our options. Acceptance frees up resources. It helps break us out of the freeze mode into whatever type of action is required. As a very simple example, imagine you are crossing the road, a horn sounds, you turn to see a bus speeding towards you. The freeze / denial response may cause you to throw out your hands, as if to stop the bus, to screw your eyes tight, as if doing that will make the bus go away. The acceptance response prompts you to use your fear to jump out of the way!

Now, denial can be used as a coping mechanism. It may be used in order to give us time to process information or come to terms with something. It may be that we need to shut something out in order to get something else done. That may mean ignoring bad behaviour in the short term in order to affect change in the long term. There are numerous examples of people ignoring major injuries in order to walk to survival, for example. In a sense, our earlier Happy Place exercise is a form of denial. So in the right context, some denial may be useful. But problems begin when that denial becomes an ingrained response.

I guess the most widespread understanding of acceptance and denial is when we talk about addictions. Most of us have heard of the Alcoholics Anonymous saying, "Hi, my name is..... and I'm an alcoholic." Recovery begins with accepting that there is a problem. But if we take a look at our everyday lives, we may find many issues that we are in real denial over.

We may constantly excuse the bad behaviour of another person. "That's just the way they are." "It's probably my fault." Some years ago I worked in a company where numerous complaints were made to management about a

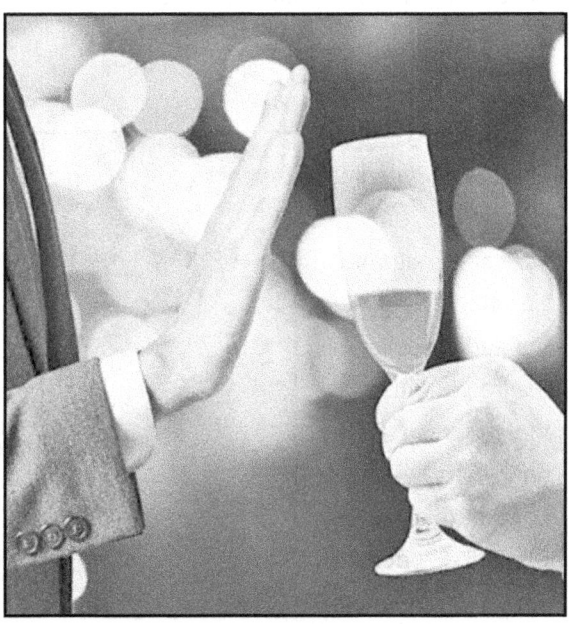

particular individual's constant inappropriate comments to younger female members of staff. The response from management was "Oh, that's just B's way, he's only being friendly." In other words, a complete denial of B's unacceptable behaviour.

We do this to ourselves, too. We might deny we are putting on weight, we might deny that we feel unwell, "No, I'm fine, I don't need to go to the doctor." My father almost died as a result of that one, he suffered for days with sharp pain and was eventually rushed into hospital with a burst appendix!

It is interesting to note that we often deny things that we do have control over, or perhaps there is a refusal to accept that our behaviour is causing or exacerbating the issue. In this case, the denial is blocking our response.

RESPOND OR REACT?

I'm talking here about our immediate response in a stressful situation. This harkens back to our earlier section on control, and the fact that *ourself* is the only thing we have control over. I say response, because, generally a response is better than a reaction. The latter ties in with our freeze, or what is called the *Startle Reflex*. This is a largely unconscious defensive reaction to a sudden stimuli - a sudden noise, a sharp movement, for example. The eyes blink, the head turns, the shoulders twitch, the hands raise up, we jump.

That is on a physical level. We can also have a Startle Reflex on a psychological or emotional level. There may be a person who knows exactly which button to press to trigger your emotional flinch. Externally, you may exhibit many of the same characteristics the flinch reaction. There's a sharp breath and in our minds we think *Oh…for eff's sake, not this again.* Our back is put up, to use a familiar, and somewhat physically accurate, term!

These are reactions, then. Much like if someone suddenly throws a ball at is, and we flinch to protects ourselves - the ball hits us and drops.

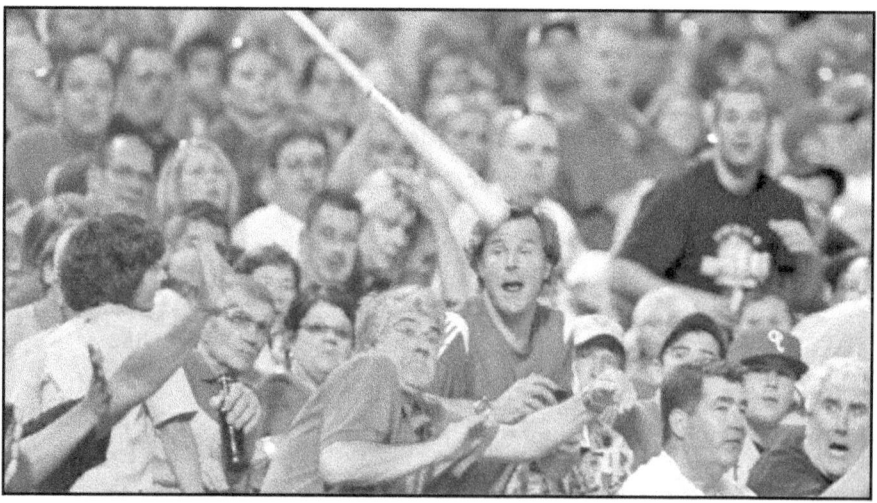

A response in the same situation is to catch the ball. In other words, a more conscious action. It may be learned, as in the case of an expert driver hitting a patch of black ice. The novice flinches and jerks the wheel, setting up a skid. The expert responds and steers smoothly into the skid, so keeping control of the car.

We can think of the same thing on a stress level. We already have some of the tools, in terms of our breathing exercises. Now, we may have to truncate them somewhat but even a quick in-breath, short hold and exhale can do the job. It buys us a second for our conscious mind to click back into place and take control of our response.

A response, then, should be more measured than a reaction and result in a more positive outcome. On hearing that the train has been delayed, a reaction may be to stamp, swear, spend the next half hour muttering angrily. A response might be to think "great, I've got more time to read my book."

PREPARATION

Knowing that we cannot control certain events brings us the option of preparing for them. On the one hand we prepare mentally, as above. On the other, we can put measures in place to help the situation. The simplest example is the weather. We are out and get caught in a downpour. Now I'm wet and miserable. A simple preparation would be to check the weather forecast and take an umbrella. Stress averted!

Wider preparation may involve getting up ten minutes earlier so you don't have to rush in the morning. It might be planning a response to a work colleague's behaviour rather than losing your temper (reaction) with them. That could mean involving other people in the situation, which brings us to our next step.

CIRCLE OF INFLUENCE

We may not have control over many things and people but we do often have some measure of influence. We can talk to others in order to help resolve personal difficulties. We can complain in various ways to a company or organisation. We can approach our elected representatives and lobby them over particular issues. In the days of social media, we have unparalleled access to a potentially huge audience. And we can also join or set up organisations, charities or pressure groups relating to issues that concern us.

So another thing to take into account, maybe as part of our preparation, is to think of that circle of influence and how we can use it in order to change a stressful situation. In the case of our work colleague's behaviour, as above, could we perhaps speak to any other people affected, then approach the colleague as a group? Or could can raise our concerns with the office manager or personnel department and have them resolve the issue?

Simply Flow

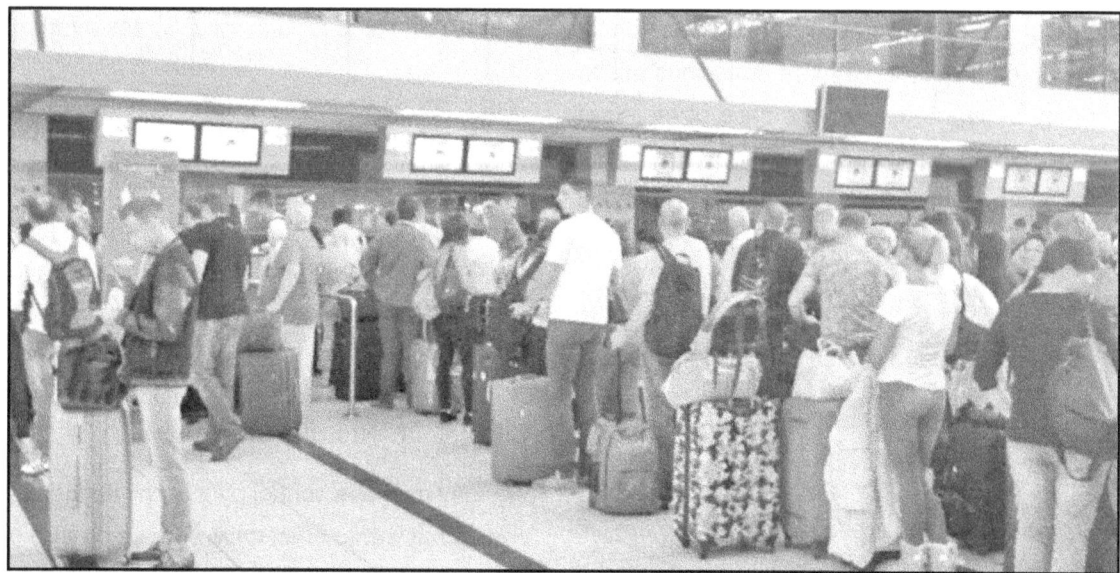

Another aspect of Influence is how our own behaviour can affect others. Think of children, they will generally copy the behaviour they grow up with, so parents should ideally be good role-models. Another way of looking at it is that if we go around being very tense, aggressive and rude to people we are likely to attract more stress into our life.

Sometimes we can feel very isolated and alone when facing difficulties. The Circle of Influence is one way of breaking out of that negative thought pattern and moving into positive action.

IN PRACTICE

Having looked at some tools for stress management, let's look at some typical situations and show how these methods could be employed within them. The beauty of the principle based approach is that once we understand the *hows and whys* of a method, we can very easily adapt it to suit the circumstances - and, as we have seen, whatever the situation, our stress response tends to be pretty much the same. So, onto some practical suggestions.

THE DELAYED FLIGHT

You are at the airport on time, ready for your flight to visit friends abroad. The announcement comes over the tannoy that your flight has been delayed for at least two hours. Perhaps more.

Response - swear (quietly!). Research has shown that swearing can actually reduce tension! If you feel yourself becoming stressed, go into a little Burst Breathing, and/or sit down and do a little Quiet Sitting.

Acceptance and control - this situation is obviously way beyond our control, so there is no choice but to accept it. No point in becoming angry, then, as we are unable to exert any influence on the flight departure time.

Circle of Influence - we could complain to the airline staff, perhaps. Calmly works best, shouting and ranting at service staff never bears fruit (however tempting it may be at times!). We might also share frustrations with our fellow passengers. It doesn't resolve anything but everyone feels better after a good group moan!

Preparation - did you bring a book? Do you have some work you can be doing on your laptop? If so, look upon the delay as an opportunity to get something done. Have a meal, do some shopping, buy something for your friends. Don't forget to text them to let them know you are going to be late.

THE JOB INTERVIEW

You are sitting in reception, waiting for your interview for a new job. You are very keen to get the job, it's a good company to work for. You've heard that the interview will likely be tough. They are running late, your interview was supposed to start fifteen minutes ago.

Response - as you are sitting and waiting, go into Quiet Sitting. Keep eyes open as you probably don't want to be nodding off!

Acceptance and control - another situation we have very little control over. We have to accept the circumstances.

Circle of Influence - perhaps you know someone who works at the company who can put a word in (if appropriate). Be polite in your dealings with the company leading up to the interview. That means in any written correspondence as well as the receptionist or anyone else you speak to on the day.

Preparation - hopefully you have prepared as much as possible for the interview. You have a clear idea of what the company does, you have a good CV that you are confident with (don't be tempted to lie or exaggerate on a CV!) and you have thought up some answers to those awkward questions beloved of interviewers!

You are on time, you look the part, you are keen and eager. Don't worry too much about appearing nervous, a good interviewer will expect some nerves. Plus you don't want to come across as arrogant or cocky.

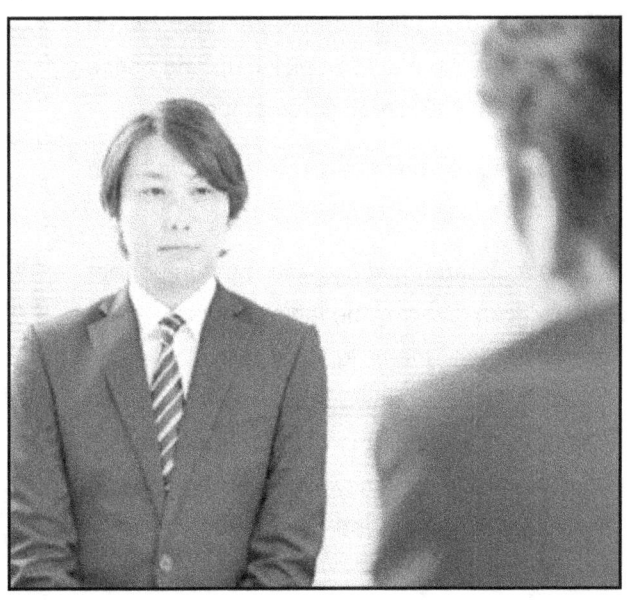

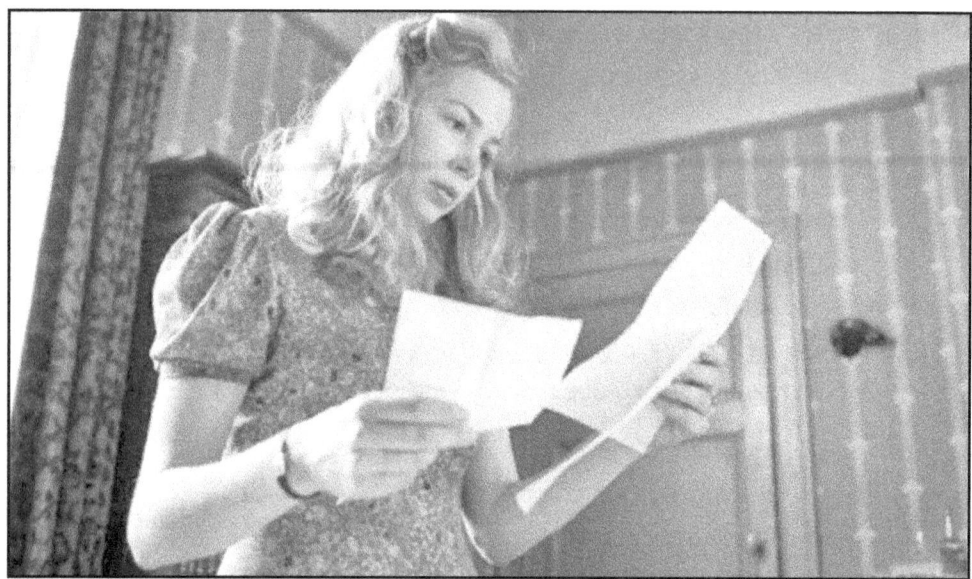

Perspective - if you don't get the job, well, there are others. Perhaps the company is not all it's cracked up to be, in any case! Keep looking, the right one will turn up soon.

THE CREDIT CARD BILL

The letterbox rattles, there's a crisp, white envelope on the mat. You pick it up and notice that it's from your credit card company.

Response - if your heart rate goes up, then work into a little Burst Breathing.

Acceptance and control - the most important advice I can give anyone facing unwanted bills is *don't ignore them!* Ignored bills do not go away, in fact they only mount up. At a certain point, if you default, the bill may may passed on to a collection agency, who will not only add their fee to your debt but may also come knocking on your door.

Circle of Influence - people sometimes hide bills or financial issues from their partner. There can be few situations where this is a good idea. Sharing problems can help not only ease our stress but the people we share with can bring another perspective or think of possible solutions you may have missed.

Preparation - if debts are building up, it is a good idea to create an income /expenditure sheet. It doesn't have to be anything fancy. Simply make a list of your monthly incomings, another of your monthly outgoings. This will give you a clear picture of what, if any, spare income you have. It will also allow your to check your outgoings, to see if there is anything you can cut back on.

Perspective - modern economies run on debt. I remember my parents saving to buy items, credit cards were largely unheard of until the

1970s. Now, almost everyone has at least one credit card, not to mention store cards, loans, mortgages and so on.

No-one should feel ashamed or embarrassed about being in debt. There are also many good resources we can turn to, from internet sites to organisations such as Citizens Advice. We should also speak directly to our creditors, they often have some kind of scheme available for those in difficulty.

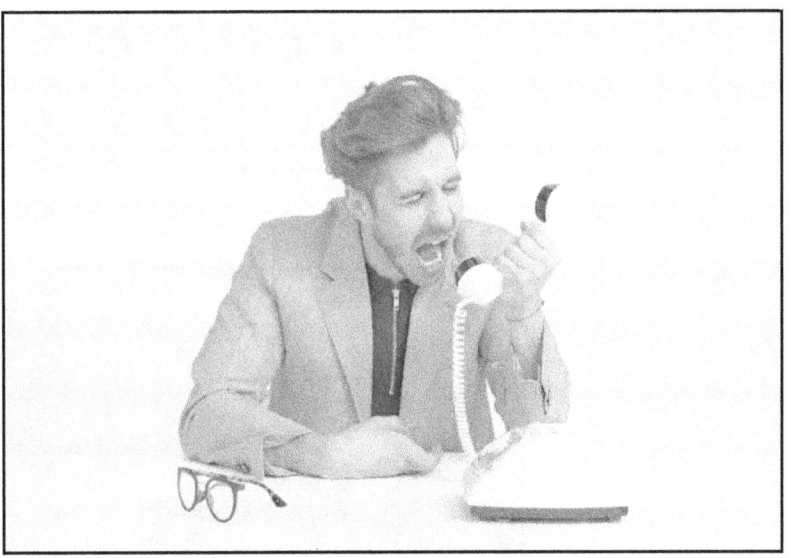

However tempting it is, I would totally avoid short-term loan merchants or, even worse, loan sharks, you will likely end up in even deeper debt.

AGGRESSIVE WORK COLLEAGUE

"Brian at the office really stresses me out. I find him a bit bullying and over-bearing, I'm starting to dread going into work."

Response - if you get upset can you remove yourself from the situation? Take a few minutes to yourself.

Acceptance and control - such behaviour is unacceptable. Understanding this should empower you into taking control of the situation.

Circle of Influence - do your other colleagues feel the same? Speak to your HR department and/or your line manager.

Preparation - log any incidents as they occur. Do not respond to any provocation, remain as calm as you can. If possible, get back up from any witnesses.

Perspective - is there a reason the person is acting this way? Stress in their own life? Prejudice? A personality clash? Understanding this may help resolve the situation.

Try not to take the aggression personally, particularly if the person is know for this type of behaviour. Is this job important to you? A transfer or change of job may not feel fair but, if you get no resolution, it may be an option.

CHAPTER FIVE
MANAGING PHYSICAL TENSION

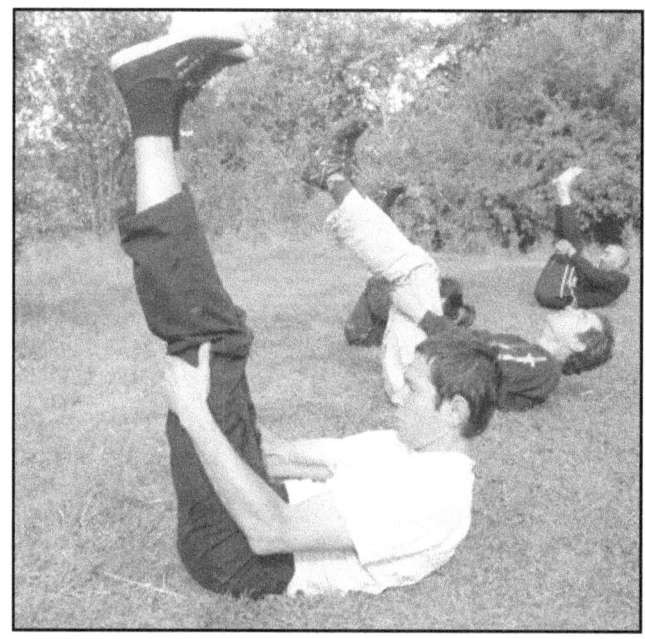

We have established that there is a strong link between mental stress and physical tension. As with our breathing, this is a two way bridge, each affects the other. This may be a hang-over from the FFF Response - we "freeze" into a defensive position, shoulders hunched, our body curled in on itself, eyes averted. Or it may be the "fight" part, our fists clench, we grimace, the chest is puffed out.

As we know, problems arise when these physical manifestations are not released. The situation has ended but the stress remains. Fortunately, there are many things we can do to counter this, especially when it comes to exercise and activities.

There are many types of exercise, and even just getting out for a good walk can help as far as stress goes. We will give you a few ideas of the types of exercise that works best for stress, as well as some other good methods for easing muscular tension. If you decide to take up any form of exercise, please be sure that it meets your abilities and needs. Don't be tempted to just go for the nearest class, or think that all types of exercise program are the same!

SELECTIVE TENSION

Muscular tension tends to be a sub-conscious response, usually to a dangerous or stressful situation. This exercise helps us to recognise tension and also to consciously control it, to switch it on and off. Having this ability means we become much more aware of tension as it takes hold, as well as giving us the ability to *breathe it away.*

You can practice this in any position - laying on your back is a good one to start with, as you can get fully comfortable. Once in position, begin Circular Breathing for a couple of minutes, allowing the body to relax.

Now we are going to introduce Selective Tension. The procedure is simple - as you inhale, the muscles tense, as you exhale they relax. The tense and relax should be in time with the breathing, which should be slow and even. When one area of the body is being tensed, the rest of the body should remain relaxed - this is selective, remember! The basic sequence runs like this:

Legs
Groin and buttocks
Abdomen
Chest
Lower back
Shoulders
Arms
Head, face, neck

Tense and relax each section in turn, for three breaths on each. Finish by tensing the whole body on the inhale, relaxing it all on the exhale (slow release) three times. Then, inhale, tense

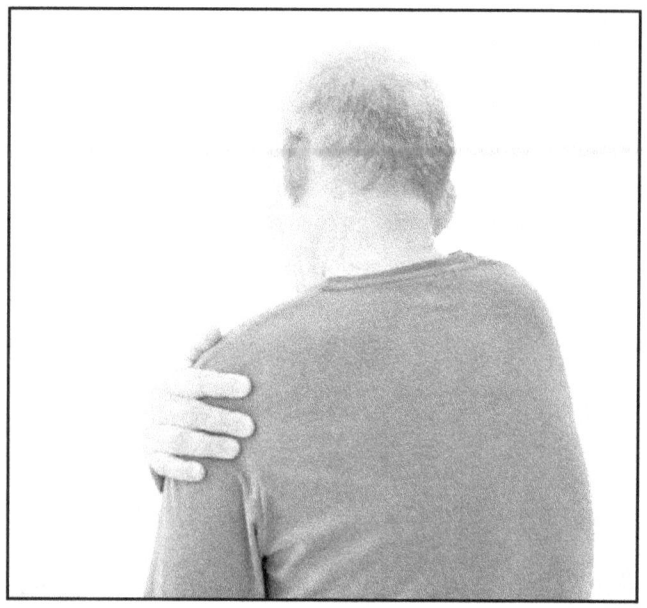

is all part of monitoring your tension throughout the day and dealing with issues as they arise.

The basic idea behind fighting tension with tension is that we overload the muscle with tension, so forcing it to relax. You can experience this by tensing your arms and fists in front of you as hard as you can, then seeing how long you can hold for. Try the same with just a little tension and you will find you can hold for much longer. The aim of this method, then, is to maximise tension in the muscle so that it is forced to relax, in the process, draining all the residual tension away.

everything again and hold the breath / tension for twenty seconds or so. Exhale, this time sharply, *pah!* and let all the tension go immediately. Spend another minute Circular Breathing, with everything relaxed. When you are ready, stretch a little and get up slowly.

Once you have the idea of this exercise, you can refine it. Rather than tense a whole limb, you might work a particular muscle group - just the calves or thighs, for example. If you have tension in a particular area, say the back, work on that place for a little longer. During the day, if you don't have time to run the full routine, pick just the body part that is giving you bother. You may be sitting at your desk and find your shoulders are tensing up. Run the Selective Tension on them a few times, hopefully it will "flush out" the tension before it can get too deep a hold. This

Another important principle with this drill is that we start conditioning the body to relax on exhalation. Think about a time you were startled or made to jump. I bet you inhaled and froze! Next time you are in that position, exhale sharply and see how it helps unlock the body, it breaks us out of that freeze response. The Russian expression is *inhale relaxes the brain, exhale relaxes the body*!

THE TENSION WAVE

The next exercise develops our ability to control and move tension. We begin in the same position as before, working our Circular Breathing for a short time. When ready, do a slow inhale and, in time with the breathing, tense the whole body from the feet up.

In other words, the tension starts in the feet and travels up the body - legs, stomach, all the way to the crown of the head. As the inhale finishes, the whole body is tense. This does not need to be deep tension, you can keep it fairly light at first. As you progress, you will gain the ability to work deeper within the body. For now, light muscular tension is fine.

Having completed the inhale, hold for a few seconds, then slowly exhale. Now the tension is released, starting at the crown of the head, finishing with the feet. Think of it as a glass filling up with water and emptying, or as a wave of tension and relaxation. Everything should be smooth and in time with the breathing.

Tense feet to head three times, then reverse direction for three times - in other words, now go inhale (tense head to feet), exhale, (relax feet to head). So, three times each way, do some normal Circular Breathing for a time, then finish as before.

MOVING TENSION

The ability to move tension through the body is a useful skill. In martial arts, we use this as a method to absorb powerful blows and strikes. It works equally well in moving tension away from a stiff shoulder and out of the hand, too! Another benefit of this exercise is that it teaches us about "movement chains" within the body, how parts of the body connect in order to transmit movement, what we refer to as Wave Movement. However that is moving away from our current topic, so, back to tension!

We are going to start by tensing the right hand into a fist. Next, tense the forearm, the upper arm and the shoulder. Maintain the tension for now, taking it across to the other side, shoulder, upper arm, forearm, left fist. At the end, both arms and shoulder are tense, all on the inhale.

Next, exhale, start to relax, left fist first, left forearm, upper arm, shoulder, then across and back down to the right fist. In effect, this is the wave tension exercise, but only across the arms.

Once you can comfortably do that, it's time for stage two. The sequence is the same, only this

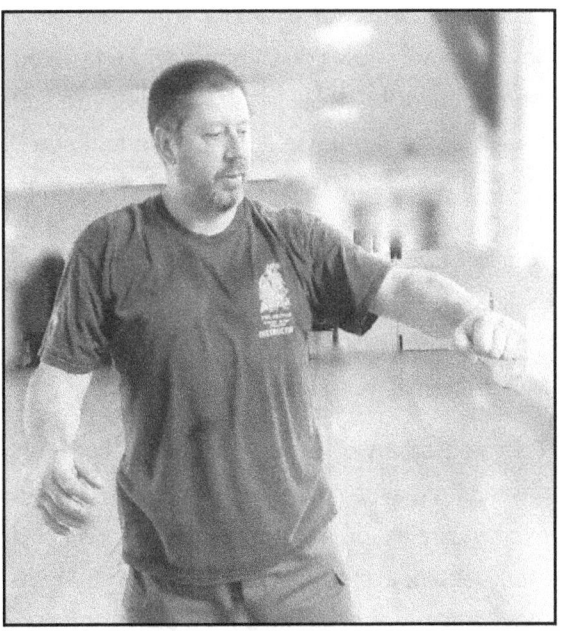

time as the forearm tenses, the fist relaxes. As the upper arm tenses, the forearm relaxes and so on. All the way across, until the left fist tenses, then relaxes, releasing the tension away. The tension, then, is moving, it passes through each muscle group without leaving anything behind.

Think of it a ball of tension that moves from the right hand to the left. The breathing pattern is inhale right fist to right chest, exhale left chest to left fist. This may take a while for you to get but stick with it. Once you have the idea, reverse the direction, left to right. You can also work the same method with the legs - foot, calf, thigh, butt and across.

Once you are able to do this, you can start to link any two points of the body together and practice moving the tension between them - right foot to left hand, for example. The ability this develops will allow you to move any unwanted tension out of the body. Let's say you have a stiff back - inhale and tense it up, exhale and see if you can "move" the tension out through the foot. This principle also works well with the sort of tension that comes from shock or fear. You can almost "shake it away" with this method.

MOVEMENT

The next area we will look at for dealing with physical stress is movement. Another Russian expression for you - *movement is the enemy of fear*. Again, this points us to the idea that we may freeze and shut down under stress.

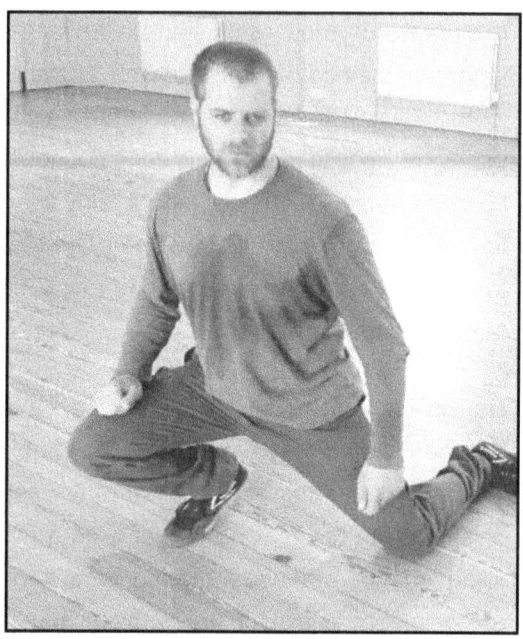

Movement helps break us out of the stress-state. As we discussed before, movement also dissipates the effects of the adrenalin dump, it flushes those chemicals out of the system.

One piece of advice, then - in the aftermath of a stressful situation, particularly where you have experienced adrenal dump, move around a bit. You may notice your hands are shaking if you try and sit still. This is your body telling you to move! Walk about a bit, jump up and down, do some type of exercise or dance movements, anything to assist with that flushing process. Of course, you can tie your breathing in with the movements too.

In terms of everyday practice, there are a number of things we can do to both help release existing tension and to help maintain our body's natural mobility and fluidity. Being relaxed (in the sense of not being rigid and stiff) in a given situation is usually far more beneficial both in informing our response to the situation and in preventing the formation of tension. At deeper levels, we can use this type of work, along with the breathing, to master our FFF response, rather than have it control us. Think, for example of a jet fighter pilot or racing car driver, who has to make split-second decisions. Imagine a heart surgeon who has to not only cut people open but then carry out extremely precise surgery, while remaining calm and detached! Just some examples that demonstrate the power of stress management!

I would highly recommend, if you don't already, that you incorporate some sort of movement routine into your stress management program. Be selective about what you choose - as I mentioned earlier, some methods will actually increase your tension. Look for intelligent, well-balanced programs, preferably ones that include some work on breathing and posture rather than ones than bombard you with noise and competition. Below I'll give you a very quick guide to the methods I use and teach to give you some ideas. More detailed. Information on these is available in our exercise books.

POSTURE

There is a strong connection between our physical and emotional postures. Think about it - when we are sad, the body tends to fold in itself, we cross our arms, the head droops. When we are on top of the world we bound out of our front door, head held high, shoulders back, smiling. This is two way link - likewise, if we have pain or injury in the body it affects our mood and emotional state.

Our general body posture and condition also has a profound effect on our heath. If we are hunched over, breathing can be compromised. Poor posture can result in various ailments. If the body became less mobile the joints stiffen up. Poor posture when moving or lifting can result in back injuries and so on.

Good posture simply means keeping the body in balance. It is not about standing to attention in a tense, military fashion but about maintaining a relaxed, neutral position,

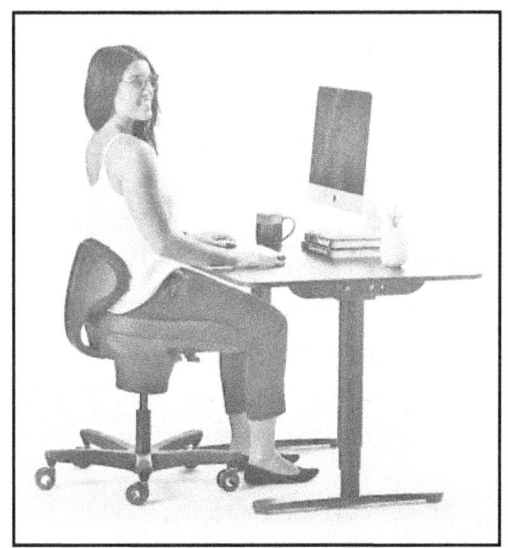

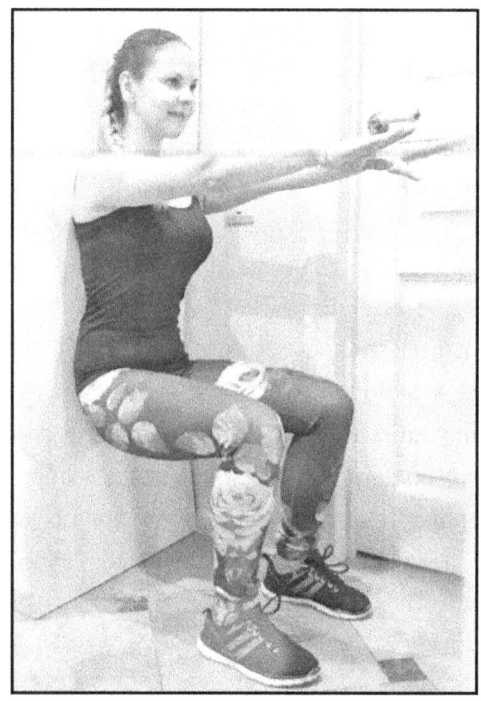

shoulders and hips level, spine straight.

You can check your posture in a mirror. Stand normally and lok to see if your shoulders tilt, and if your hips are level. When you sit, try and keep the back upright and don't let the head sag forward or back, this can cause tension in the neck. It is very good to get into the habit of monitoring your posture regularly throughout the day. If you are sitting at a desk for a long period of time, every now and then check that you are not hunching, leaning, or tilting the neck, for example. You might find a back or foot support helps, or even a specialised posture chair.

A great exercise for improving posture is the Assisted Squat. Find a secure, flat surface, such as a wall or a closed door. Stand with your back to it. Bring the feet away from the wall a little and to a comfortable position, usually just over shoulder width apart. The toes must point in the same direction as the knees. They may be pointing straight forward, or be turned out a little, though not pointing inwards.

Inhale, then on an exhale, slowly bend the knees a little and lower yourself down. Just go to your comfortable range of motion. The trick is to maintain the alignment of the body, so the back should remain in full contact with the supporting surface, from shoulders to tailbone. If you tuck the tailbone in a little and tilt the pelvis slightly, you will find it more comfortable.

Hold for a while as you inhale, exhale and when ready slowly straighten up again. Holding this position for a few minutes will help with posture, strengthen the legs and also help to relax the hips - but take it steady, it can be quite demanding on the legs!

JOINT ROTATION

Excepting injury or illness, there is no reason for us to be less mobile when we age as we were as youngsters. The problem is that we often "forget to move." We get fixed into very particular movement patterns, we lose our natural freedom. Think of how children move - they crawl, run, walk, roll, climb. Their movement tends to be totally unselfconscious, with very much a playful or exploratory mindset. Contrast that with an older person who sits all day at work, sits in the car on the way home, sits in the armchair watching TV of an evening. Ask them to run or clamber around things and they will find it very difficult. Not because they can't but because they have forgotten how to!

To some extent playing sports can get around this issue, though with many sports comes the risk of injury. Fortunately there any many other forms of exercise to choose from. If you don't have time to take any of these up, try and build a regular Joint Rotation routine into your life. This simply means slowly working through every joint in the body and rotating it as much as you can.

As a guide sequence, start with the head. Drop the chin forward to the chest, then slowly begin to rotate the head clockwise. After a few circles, stop and change direction. Make sure the shoulders are relaxed, make sure you go slow. If your neck is stiff, work only to your comfortable range of motion. Don't attempt to force anything.

Follow the same procedure down into the shoulders - lift and drop them, then rotate. Keep your breathing natural and slow. From the shoulders you can work into elbows and hands. Then try rotating your trunk. Expand and relax the chest. Wave the spine like a belly dancer. Circle the hips. Finally, work down into the legs. You can use a support and stand on one leg. Lifting the other, rotate the ankle, knee and hip, in both directions.

That whole routine need only take five minutes. Not only will it relax you, it will keep all your joints "oiled" and help you in monitoring your physical state.

FLOOR MOVEMENT

We mentioned children earlier. Think of how toddlers move on the floor - crawling, rolling, stretching. If you have a suitable space, spend some time on the ground. At first, just try rolling from side to side. Imagine the body as a

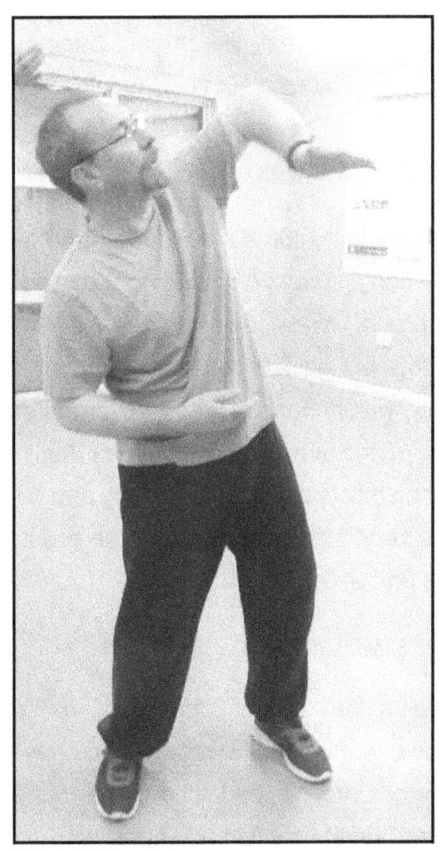

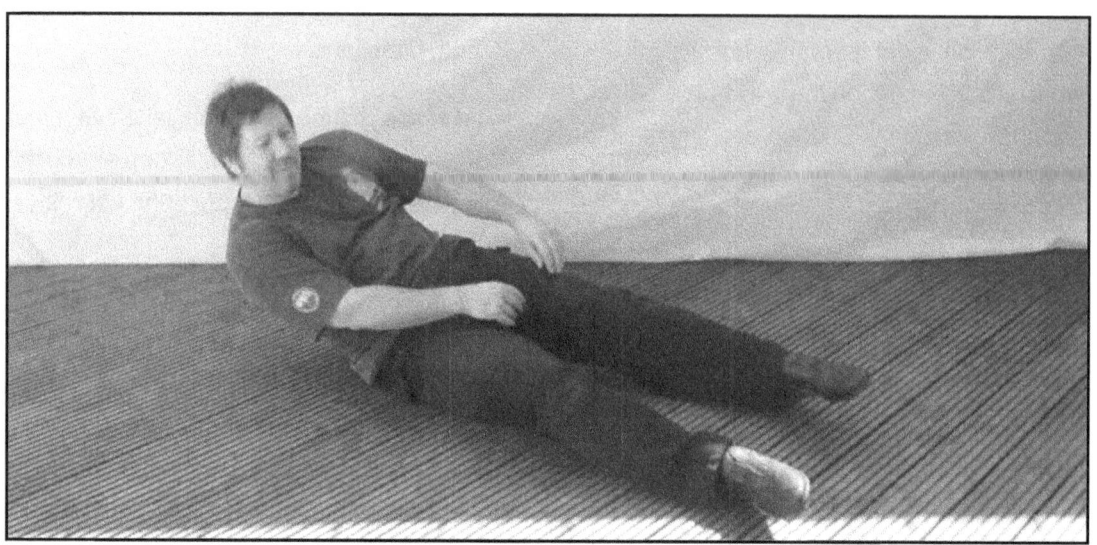

cylinder. Lift the hands and feet and allow the body to roll. Next, lay on your back and try to move just by rotating your shoulders. Then try the same thing using other parts of the body - the arms, the legs, etc.

You could try some breakdance type moves, or you can just work on going from seated position to prone. When ready you can even practice falling - I advise you do this under qualified supervision! Each of these movements will help free up the body, working not only Joint Rotation but also core strength, breathing and relaxation. it is very difficult to move on the ground if you are tense!

FREE MOVEMENT

Apply the same principles to standing movements. Turn the radio up and have a bit of a dance around the kitchen! The trick is to not worry about how it looks. Go slow, but explore how your body can move in so many different directions. How you can change height, how you can flow from one movement to the next. This is the sort of feeling that dancers and martial artist strive for, to be truly present in the moment, lost in the flow of movement. It is a powerful therapy for both body and mind.

Try and be aware in your daily life of movement habits. If you sit a lot of the time, set an alarm to beep once an hour. On that beep, get up and walk around a bit, do some stretches, have a quick run up the stairs. Watch how you carry things. I had a friend who suffered from a frozen shoulder in her twenties. The doctor worked out that she had been carrying a heavy handbag over that shoulder and constantly hunched it up, even when not carrying the bag.

Keep an eye on how you walk, how you sit - along with monitoring breathing and tension, this will soon become a natural part of your everyday life. Many people mask their body's discomfort, or say that any aches and pains caused are just "part of getting older." Nonsense! Mobility is the key to good health in later life, and the key is in your hands.

STRETCHING

Stretching is a very natural activity, it's often the first thing we do on waking up in the morning. Animals stretch frequently and quite naturally - people should do the same! Some equate stretching with extreme flexibility but our approach is to use stretching as tension release. We strongly advise slow moving and static stretching rather than the "bouncing" or ballistic type, which can cause problems with the tendons and ligaments.

The slow moving stretch is the kind we do everyday. We have a bit of a stiff back so we put our hands on our hips and rotate the trunk, for example. We will add in breathing to the movement - an inhale as we ready, then an exhale on the stretch. Remember, the exhale is to help the muscles relax.

Pick a comfortable movement to start - reaching the hands up in the air, say. Stand in neutral position, inhale. As you exhale, reach up with the hands. Inhale back to the start position.

A static stretch is the same but rather than return to the start position, we hold the stretch for a period of time. Around 30 seconds is okay to start. Once again, keep the muscles relaxed. Sometimes it helps to hold the stretched limb in place. If the muscle feels particularly tense, you can use burst breathing to help relax it. In any case, do not hold the breath while you hold the stretch!

There are more advanced forms of stretching, such as the Russian Stretch but these basic methods will get you started. Incorporate them into your daily routine. You can do some while sat a desk, or you could bend and touch your toes while waiting for the kettle to boil. Keep your movements simple. Once you get the idea

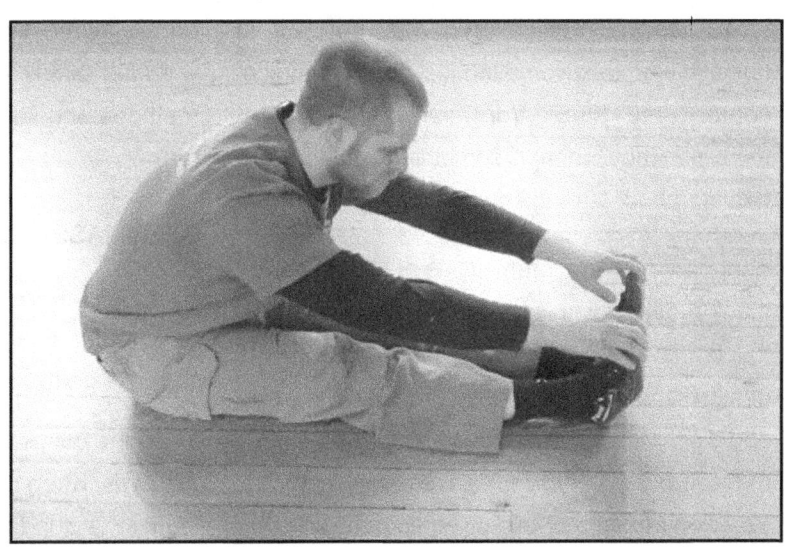

you can try more challenging stretching positions (see our *Fitness Over 40* or other sources). The important thing is that you take your time, never rush or bounce a stretch. The aim is to release tension not "elongate" the ligaments. Little and often is good, you will be surprised how much tension can be released with a good stretch.

MASSAGE

Massage is probably the oldest form of healing. It is such a natural thing - a parent will soothe their child through massage, we rub our temples when we have a headache and so on. Good massage brings benefits on many levels. It relaxes muscles, aids posture, and restores the skeletal system to its proper form. Massage can also stimulate blood circulation and the lymphatic system and aid with soft tissue damage.

It was recently discovered that patients in hospital who received even just a minor level of contact and touch from carers had faster recovery times. There is something soothing and healing about "caring contact."

There are many different styles of massage and many methods within those. For the purpose of this book we will take you through two routines designed to help with stress; a self-massage and a similar partner massage sequence. These massages are very simple, every day"methods. You don't need any oils or equipment and you

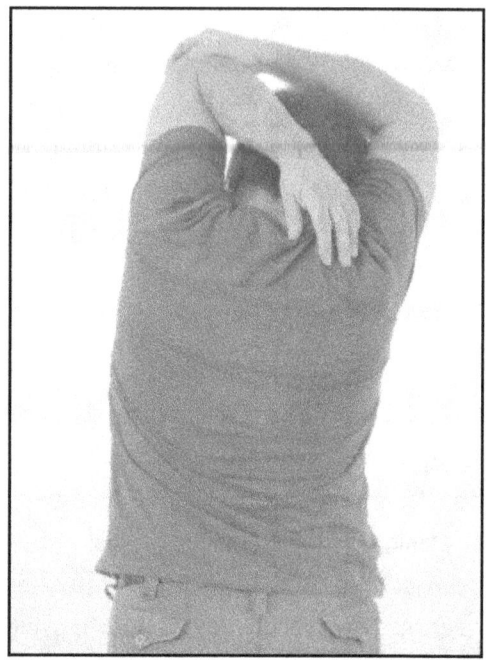

can do them anywhere a person can sit down.

They are gentle methods and so should not cause any issues but our usual medical caveats apply. Be aware of your own medical issues and double aware if massaging another person. We will also briefly discuss some other massage methods should you wish to explore this area further.

SELF MASSAGE

Sit down and run through a couple of minutes of Circular Breathing. Then rub your hands briskly together to generate heat in the palms.

Once the palms are warm, place the palms over the eyes. Keep the eyes open, allow the heat to "sink in" around the eyes.

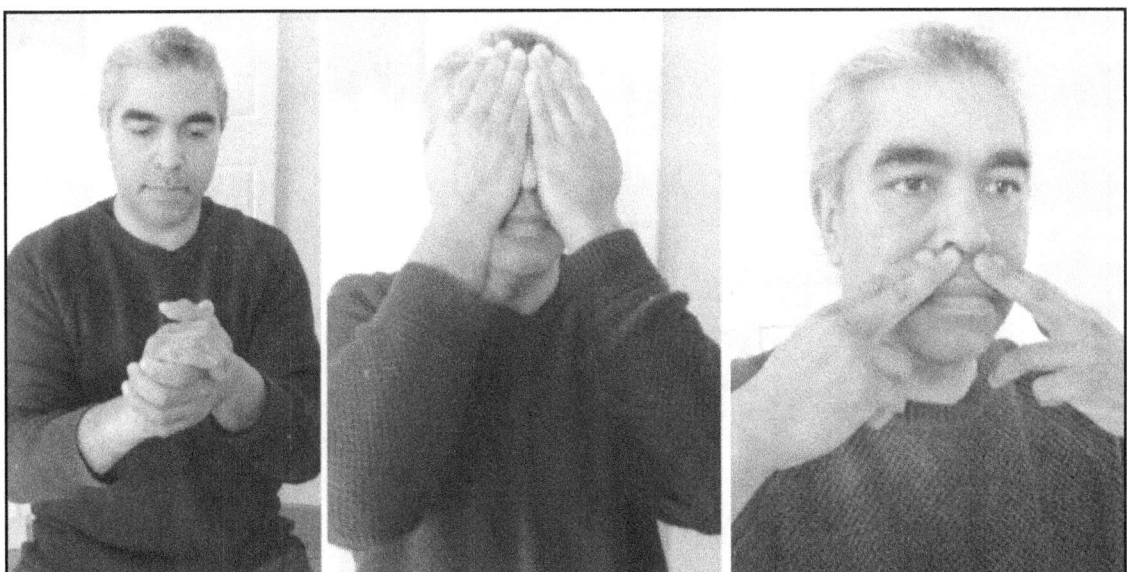

Now, using the fingertips, start to gently press and massage around the eyes. Do not put too much pressure on the eyes themselves. Work under the eyebrow ridge, into the corners, and underneath the eyes. There are many small muscles in this area that hold a lot of tension, so take your time with this part of the massage.

Bring the fingers up to the temples. Press and make small circles, working into the muscle. Again, be sensitive to the amount of pressure you need - too little achieves nothing, too much may create more stress.

Work up onto the forehead, making small circles. Work along the scalp line and back out again, then a little lower down across the forehead itself.

Next, place the fingers in the corner of the eyes and work down the sides of the nose, applying light pressure. This will help with any sinus issues.

Rub out onto the cheeks and across the top lip. Sweep out to just in front of the ears and massage the jaw hinge. There is often a lot tension stored here.

Rub the palms briskly together again, then place over the ears. Feel the heat working into the muscles. Massage all around the ear, inside and out.

Place fingers under the earlobes and work from here down under the jaw line to the point of the chin. Return to earlobes and repeat a couple more times.

Next, rub the hands together again, then "wash" the whole face with the palms.

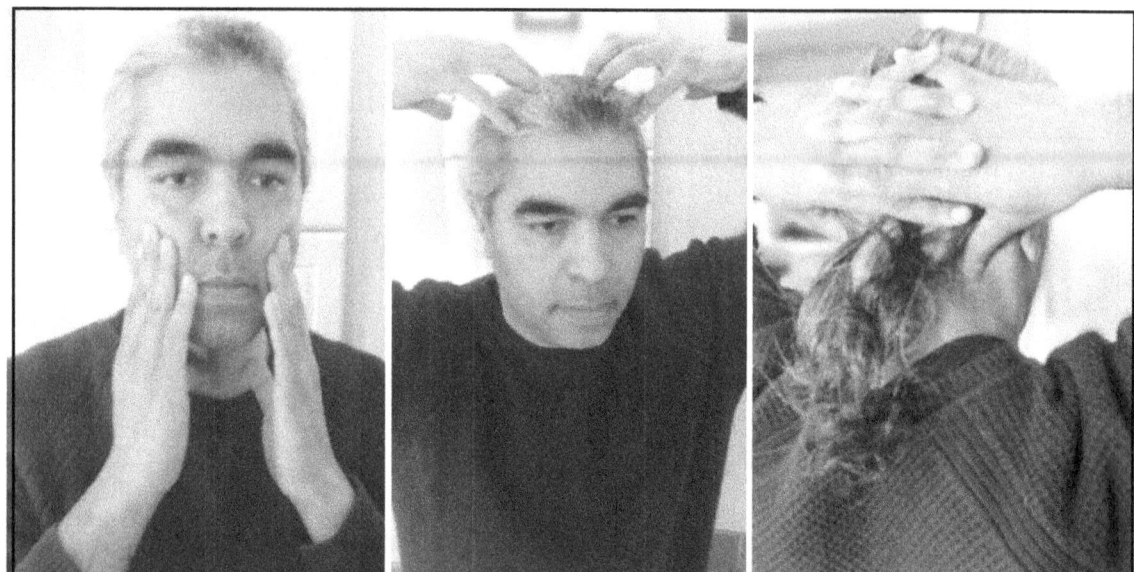

Now we start to tap the scalp. Place the hands above the head and lightly tap with the fingertips. Start at the crown and work down and back. Then return to the crown and go down the sides. Finally, from the crown again, work forwards.

Link the fingers together and place the hands on the back of the head, so that the thumbs rest at the top of the neck. Applying pressure, run the thumbs down the large muscles at the back of the neck. Lift and repeat a few times.

Place your right hand on your left shoulder. You can support it at the elbow, if you like. Massage into the muscles of shoulder and neck with a "kneading" motion. Repeat on the right shoulder.

Vigorously rub the arms, chest and stomach with the palms. Rub the thighs, all around the knees and the calves in the same way. Have a little breathe and stretch, then get up and resume your day!

PARTNER MASSAGE

Have your partner sit on a stool or a chair. Stand behind them. Start by briskly rubbing your hands together to build up heat in the palms. Once they are hot, rest the palms lightly on your partner's shoulders and both run through a minute or so of Circular Breathing.

Next, start feeling across the neck and shoulders to see which areas need the most attention. From there, rub the shoulder muscles briskly with the palm, from the neck outwards.

Start gently kneading into the shoulder muscles with your thumbs. Check with your partner to make sure you are not applying too much pressure. An option is to use the side of your hands to lightly "chop" across the shoulders.

From here, massage both sides of the neck with

the fingertips. Stand on the left side of the person and place your right hand on the back of their neck. Now place your left palm against the forehead to gently keep it in place. Spread the right hand thumb and fingers to cup the base of the skull. Glide down the back of their neck while applying light pressure. Bring the hand back to the start point when you reach the base of the neck. Repeat as required.

From the same position, holding the the forehead and base of the skull, slowly tilt the head forward. There should be no forcing, no strain. Hold for at least ten seconds, then, gently lift the head back to vertical position. Repeat a few times. After that, do the same movement but this time gently tilting the head backwards.

From there, stand behind your partner and place your left hand on their left shoulder. Use your right hand to gently push their head to the right while pushing lightly down with your left hand. Repeat on each side a few times.

Next, stand behind the person, place your hands on each side of their head. Using your fingertips, make light circular motions across the scalp. Work from back to front and then front to back. You can repeat this motion a few times. You can also repeat using the tapping movement from the solo massage routine.

From the same position, place the fingers of both hands onto the forehead. Make small circles, moving out to the temples, applying light pressure. After about ten seconds, move back up to their forehead and repeat the process a few times.

Finish the massage by briskly rubbing the shoulders a few times, then rest the hands in the very first position on the shoulders again for another couple of minutes of Circular Breathing.

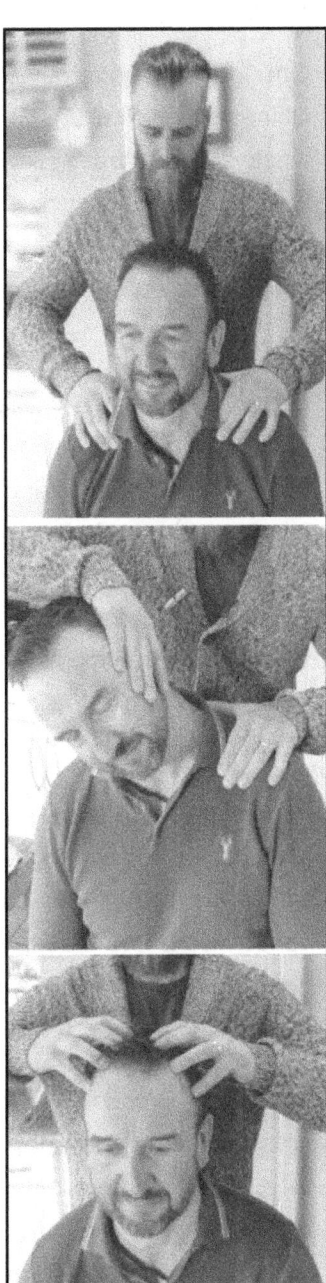

ACUPRESSURE

One of the central theories of Traditional Chinese Medicine (TCM) is that the body's innate energy (*chi* or *qi*) flows in channels called meridians. At certain points, these meridians can be accessed, either to heal (acupuncture, acupressure) or to harm (pressure points.)

Chi is said to have many sources. There is the energy we are born with, our life-force. On top of that, we gain chi from breathing, from food, from our environment and from exercise (*chi kung* or *qigong*). Modern medical science fails to recognise many of the claims of TCM, despite which it has spread around the world - acupuncture treatments are available on the NHS, for example. In China it remains widely practiced alongside Western forms of medicine.

Acupressure is just one method of accessing acupuncture points without needles. It is a very simple practice that we can use to help with stress levels. It is a deep subject in itself but here we will give you just a few main points that you can try out for yourself.

The normal procedure is to apply appropriate pressure to the relevant point, or to press or massage it in a certain way. We can apply to ourselves, or to another person, and many of these points can easily be incorporated into our earlier massage routines. We press with the thumb or fingertips and it should be a firm pressure, working into the point. You'll get the feel with a little practice.

Hand Valley Point
Situated in the webbing between your thumb and index finger. Stimulating this point is said to reduce stress, headaches, and neck pain. Use your index finger and thumb to apply pressure to the point of your other hand.

Massage for a minute or so, taking slow, deep breaths.

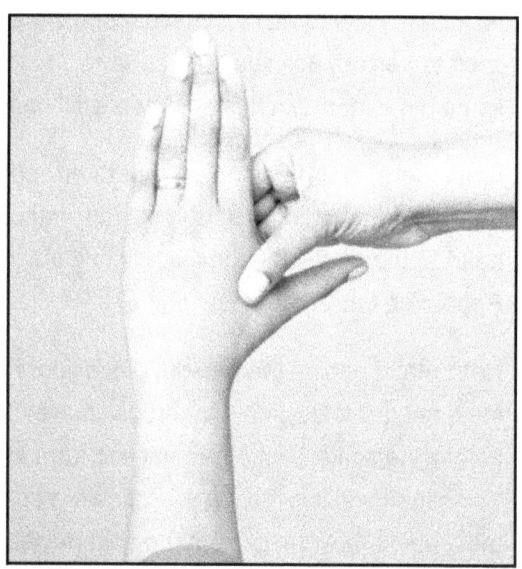

Shoulder Well Point
Situated at the top of the shoulder muscle. Relieves stress, muscle tension, and headaches. It is also said to induce labour, so don't use this point if you're pregnant.

To find it, pinch your shoulder muscle with your middle finger and thumb. Apply gentle, firm pressure with your index finger and massage the point.

Don't Worry!

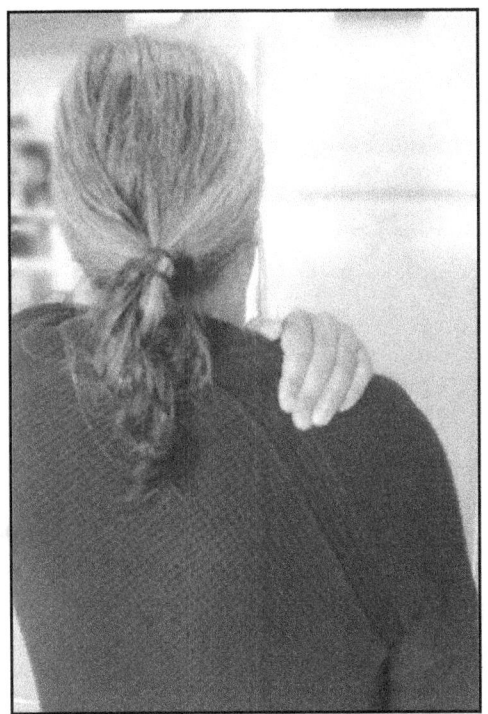

Temple Point

Situated at the temple, in the depression just lateral to the outer end of the eyebrow.

This is a nice point for the treatment of headaches and migraine headaches, especially those related to sinus conditions. Use the ends of your first and middle fingers. With light contact, move your fingers in small, circular motions. The circle should be lifting up backwards, going down forwards. Apply to the left and right sides simultaneously, continuing for two to three minutes, or longer.

So, there we have three very simple to use acupressure points that will help relieve some common minor ailments. Let's next look at working deeper into the the muscles

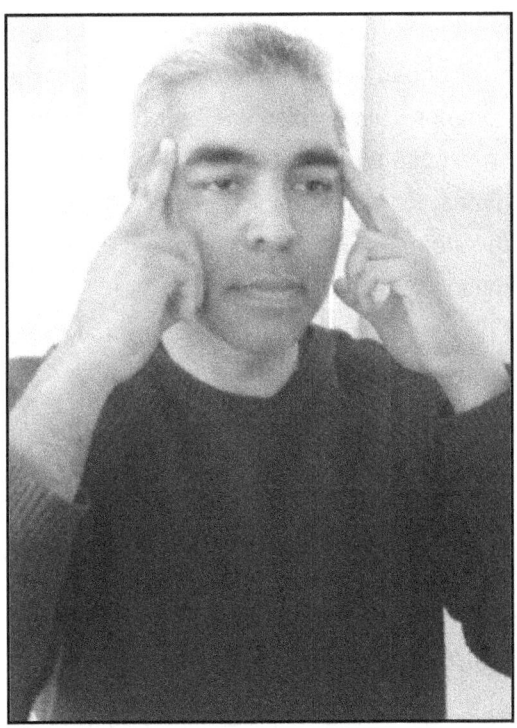

TRIGGER POINT MASSAGE

Did you ever feel like you have a "knot" in your muscle? The technical term for these are *myofascial trigger points*. They are tight balls of overworked fibres in the muscles, similar to a spasm that has been unable to release. If not treated they can cause stiffness, soreness and impede the correct function of the muscles. They may even restrict blood flow or pinch on nerves, causing sciatic type pain.

Trigger Point Massage is a great way to get relief from knots. It allows the fibres to separate and so brings blood, oxygen and nutrients to the area, as well as helping any additional toxins to drain away.

Most minor trigger points are self-treatable. It is safe, cheap, and reasonable self-help for many common pain problems. First of all, locate the sore point with your fingers. Now press on it directly or apply small, circular strokes for a minute or so. If you can, stroke parallel to the muscle fibres.

The pressure should be firm enough to be uncomfortable but not excruciating. Use Burst Breathing to assist. Work for about thirty seconds at first. Once used to it, you can work a little longer, or until the knot has eased. Should any other issues or symptoms arise, get them checked out by your doctor.

EQUIPMENT

There are a few simple items we can use to help with massage, particularly Trigger Point. A hard rubber ball is great for working into tense muscles. Roll it on the floor with the sole of your foot, or sit and use it along the muscles of your calf and thigh.

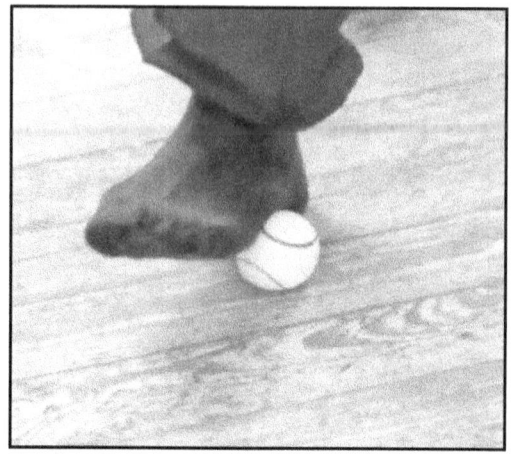

A larger ball can work the same for the back muscles. Simply place your weight on it and roll slightly.

You can use a short stick to work into the long muscles in the body, particularly the legs and abdomen. Apply firm pressure as your brush the stick along the muscle length. This will also work nicely as a partner massage into the shoulders. Remember to avoid contact with the joints / bone.

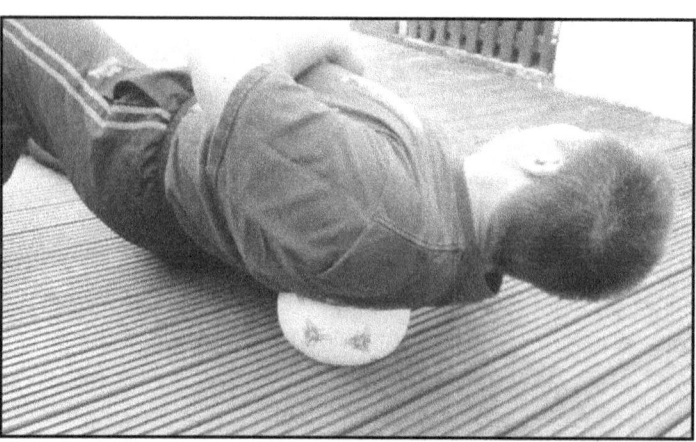

Foam rollers are readily available and come in different sizes. Use a smaller one in the same way as the ball. Get a larger one to work your back. To use, lay across the roller and use your bodyweight to apply moderate pressure to a specific muscle or muscle group. Next, roll slowly, no more than an inch per second. When you find

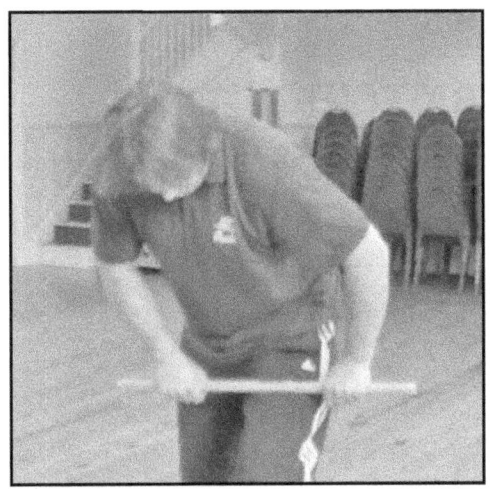

areas that are tight, pause for several seconds and relax as much as possible. Remember your breathing! You should slowly start to feel the muscle releasing, and the pain lessen.

If a spot is too painful to apply direct pressure, shift the roller and apply pressure on the surrounding muscles. Work to relax the whole area, then go back to the original spot.

You can also use the roller for the limbs, working on the floor or a hard surface such as a table top.

If you don't have a foam roller, you can use a large, plastic drinks bottle. Fill it with warm water and use as a roller - be sure the top is on tight!

You may find the use of oils beneficial in some massage, with the added bonus of soothing scents with aromatherapy oils (be sure to use decent oils and dilute appropriately.)

One last piece of equipment is a massage chair. You may find these helpful in some circumstances. These are usually in the form of a chair back with revolving balls that you lean back into. They can be pricey but the best ones can give a surprisingly good massage. Perhaps try before you buy?

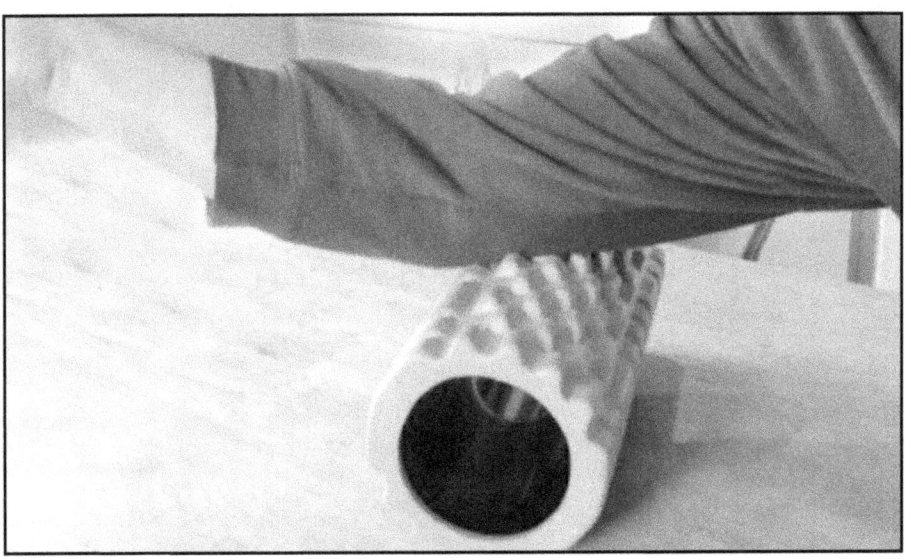

CHAPTER SIX
LIFESTYLE STRATEGIES

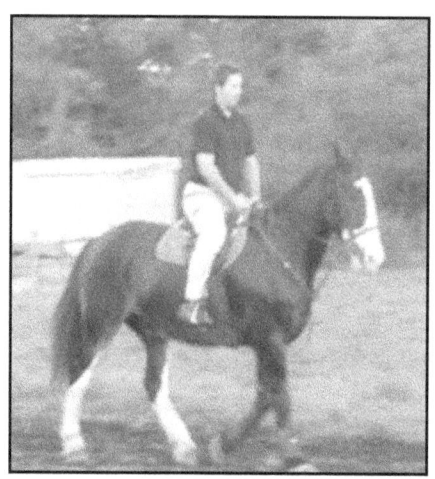

Stress rarely arises in isolation and can be exacerbated by many other factors. Similarly, stress is rarely confined to a single event, and will have wider repercussions, spreading its influence into all our other activities. How, then, can we take steps to ensure that these wider effects are lessened? Are there strong coping mechanisms that we can put into place? Do we also need to examine different parts of our overall lifestyle to see if there are areas we can tweak in order to make us more "stress-resistant?"

COMPENSATION ACTIVITIES

This term was coined by Bolivian philosopher Oscar Ichazo (b 1931) as just one aspect of his much wider body of work (which became the foundation for the Arica School, a human potential movement group founded in 1968.)

Ichazo described these as activities that we turn to in order to escape from or to mask our feelings of stress and tension. They may be very specific activities, or they may be certain types of behaviour or mindset. These compensations tend to be negative, and may well have a detrimental effect on other aspects of our lives.

If they become habitual responses to stressful situations, the compensations can become problems in themselves, leading us into a downward spiral. The stressful situation leads to the negative compensation, which, in turn results in more stress and so on.

Ichazo categorised and listed these compensations as follows:

1. Toximania - the use of cigarettes, alcohol, drugs

2. Psychosomatic Illness - person becomes preoccupied with health, perhaps even to the point of hypochondria

3. Over-exertion - immersion into a particular activity, such as over-work, excessive exercising.

4. Crime - it might be low-level, such as shoplifting, it may be plotting to or actually causing harm against a perceived "enemy"

5. Phobia - ranging from dislike to a very strong aversion

6. Panic - anxiety attacks, unable to make decisions

7. Gluttony - excessive intake of food or drink or even more abstract things, such as spending all day watching soap operas!

8. Cruelty - abusive behaviour and language, physical harm, violence

9. Sensuality - excessive or extreme sexual activity

Ichazo also assigned three levels to these mechanisms. If we take alcohol as an example, then the three levels would be:

Temporary - having a couple of drinks at the end of a hard week

Every day - using alcohol as an anesthetic to *take the edge off*

Addiction - unable to drink without getting drunk.

If we read through the list above, I imagine there's few of us who could claim never to have done any of those things! And this is something that is important to realise - if your coping mechanism to a relationship break up is a big tub of ice cream and a couple of nights watching rom-coms, that's okay! Problems arise when the coping mechanism becomes the standard mode of behaviour. We all get short-tempered now and then but if our stress is causing us to be constantly vile and abusive to the people around us, then there is a problem that needs to be addressed.

THE COMPENSATION JOURNAL

If you think this is an area you need to examine in your life, then we can make a simple addition to our Trigger Journal from the earlier chapter. Once you've been keeping the basic journal for a couple of weeks and can start to identify your triggers, modify it in the following way:

What stressed me - a simple description of the event

How did I feel - a few words describing your immediate feelings

How did I compensate - what behaviour did you indulge in to counter the above

Underlying belief - what did you think about yourself?

We give some examples in the table opposite. Once again, after a couple of weeks, you can hopefully start to recognise patterns in your behaviour. You may also start to see patterns in your belief system. For example, do you often feel that you are not up to the task in hand? Or that there is something wrong with your size or appearance? This then gives us two steps to work on - our belief and our approach.

BELIEF REALITY CHECK

How true is your belief? Examine the belief to see if it holds up to scrutiny. Ask yourself four questions.

1. Is the belief true?
2. Is it realistic?
3. What is the evidence for this belief?
4. Is it helpful?

If we take the "kids" example, where the belief is that you are a terrible parent, it may run like this.

1. No, I actually devote a lot of time to my kids.
2. All kids act up at some time, and there's no such thing as a perfect parent!
3. Generally my kids are very well behaved.
4. Not really. Thoughts like that just depress me and push me into compensation behaviour.

STRESS EVENT	FEELINGS	COMPENSATION	BELIEF
Didn't finish work report on time	Embarrassed	Four pints at lunchtime	Not good enough for the job
Kids misbehaving this morning	Irritated	Swore at the kids	I'm a terrible parent
Parents won't take my advice	Frustrated	Ate a whole box of chocs	They don't take me seriously
Turned down for bank loan	Angry	Went shopping on-line	I have no control over my life

A BETTER APPROACH

The second step is to then establish a better approach to dealing with the situation. This means setting yourself a goal and a way of achieving it. Let's stick with the parenting example.

Goal - to be able to deal with the kids better in the morning

How to achieve - get up a little earlier. Have the kids lunches prepared the night before. Also, be prepared for the odd tantrum and don't take then personally.

The goal should be realistic and achievable. It could be as simple as setting your alarm clock fifteen minutes earlier, as in the above example. It could be far more complex, in which case break it down into smaller chunks.

Remember, half the battle is to be moving in the right direction! In some cases, this process might mean you enlisting the help of friends, family or work colleagues. If the issue revolves around your job, for example, perhaps you could speak to your line-manager about workloads or receiving extra training. If it's a family issue, perhaps your partner or a friend could help out with things.

This approach should go some way to obviating the need for compensatory behaviours. Without the triggering stress, there should be no need for those drinks at lunchtime, for example. However, there will still be situations where stress strikes, so let's now look at positive coping mechanisms.

COPING MECHANISMS

These are another form of compensation behaviour, but this time are activities that will have a more positive impact on our lives.

Exercise - there are myriad forms, find one which suits you best

Hobby - knitting, playing music, collecting stamps, fixing up motorbikes

Education - learn a new language, take an evening class

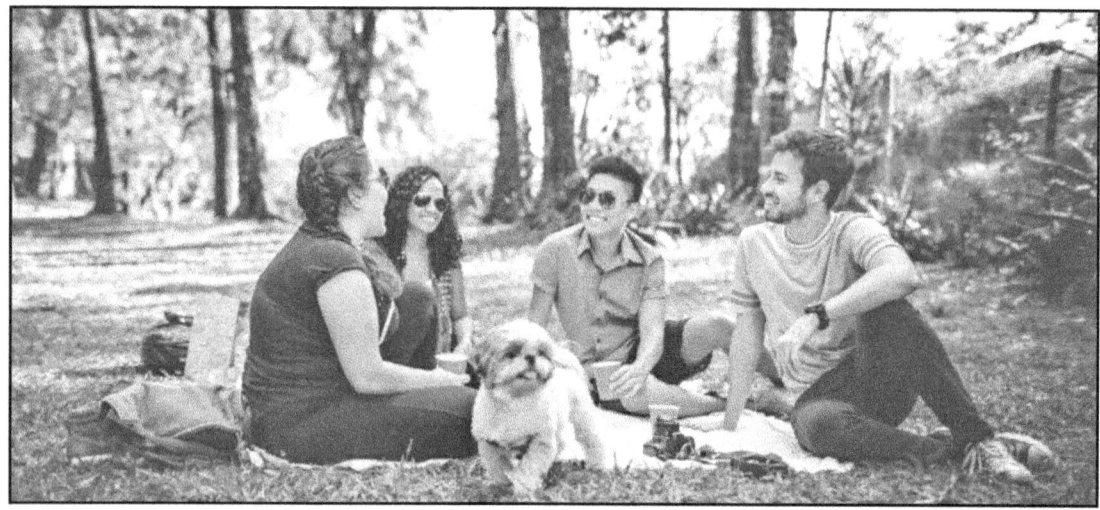

Emotional release - it's okay to show emotion! In a suitable setting, let your emotions out. Watch a sad film and cry, or a comedy to help you laugh. If you are angry, swear and punch a cushion. Let it out!

Solitude - read a book, listen to your favourite music, have a long soak in a warm bath

Socialise - meet up with some friends, go for a meal, have a good chat

Get back to nature - take a walk in the woods, or a stroll around the park, do some gardening

Be creative - try your hand at painting, do some crafting, sing a song!

I suppose each of these may also be open to excess - we may run off and become a hermit, for example! However, generally speaking, any of these activities can go a long way to helping us maintain a healthy outlook on life. One other thing, don't put off implementing these changes.

You don't have to do everything at once but if, for example, you decide you'd like to learn Spanish, then find a local course and book it up! I'm a musician and I so often hear "Oh, I always wanted to play the piano!" My answer is always the same: "Then why don't you?"

A friend of mine got so fed up with his wife saying she wanted to learn guitar, that he eventually told her "You've been saying this for three years. If you had started guitar lessons when you first said, you'd now have three years experience behind you. So do it, or stop talking about it!" Okay, so he spent a few nights sleeping on the sofa but he made a valid point!

TIME MANAGEMENT

Whoever and wherever we are, there are only so many hours in a day. Most of us tend to fall into or develop routines that revolve around our needs to sleep, work, eat and so on. How we manage our time in order to get all our tasks done is very important, yet is something, in my experience, that people rarely look at. Most of just try and "muddle through" as best we can, without ever examining how we spend our time.

Time management is the ability to plan and control how we spend the hours in our day to effectively accomplish our goals. Technology has been a great assistance in this, of course. I can remember my Grandmother having to hand wash clothes, then put them through the wringer. Nowadays, you pop them in the washing machine, job done! On the other hand, we are now attached to world 24/7 via our various devices and people expect instant answers to messages. We can watch TV or go shopping 24/7. We are in danger of losing touch with the natural rhythms of nature.

So, the first step is to determine how we are spending our time. There are apps you can get to help with this, or if you are old school, a pen and paper will do. You could even combine this with the previous journals. Your list doesn't have to be detailed, just a note of how long you spend doing what, like so:

SATURDAY
8.00 - get up, exercise, shower, breakfast
9.00 - mow the lawn and tidy up garden
10.30 - cup of tea, read paper
11.00 - go online, Facebook, e-mails
12.30 - lunch
1.15 - go to post office and supermarket
3.00 - unpack shopping, cup of tea, watch TV
4.30 - go online, check e-mail, watch youtube
6.00 - cook dinner
7.00 - watch TV
10.30 - go online, Facebook, e-mails, youtube
11.30 - bed

Another method would be to simply list the amount of time you spend in an activity. You will soon build up a picture of how you spend your time - and be honest with your reporting! In the example above, you might be surprised to find that you've spent five hours on your computer. It's probably the biggest time-thief of all!

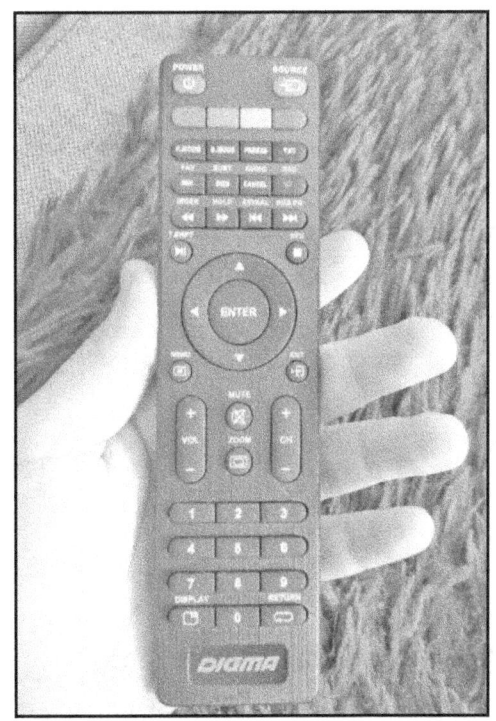

Once we have our "time audit" we can begin to make changes. There are two main approaches to this. The first is to cut your time down into chunks and assign these to specific tasks. For example, you might plan out your Saturday like this. Let's assume you are active for fifteen hours:

Housework/gardening - 2 hours
Exercise - 30 minutes
Social media - 1 hour
Cooking, eating - 2 hours
Shopping - 2 hours
Phone calls, etc - 45 minutes
Watching TV - 3 hours

Already, just by restricting your on-line time, you have a few spare hours. Of course, you have to be strict with yourself. Use a timer or alarm clock so there's no excuse to lose track of time!

I use this method to organise my work time. I'm self-employed and work from home. So while my commute is walking across the landing to the office, it does also mean that I have a lot of distractions around me and am also entirely responsible for organising myself! For me it is very tempting to spend time doing only the things that I enjoy. I hate admin and accounts, so actively have to set time slots aside in order to do those things. Meanwhile, I could do video editing or music recording all day - and into the night too!

To help, I assign myself a time limit for each job. If I spend two hours editing, I then have to spend an hour on admin, for example. I also make sure to factor in breaks away from the computer, even if its just five minutes per hour.

Now, as the saying goes, no plan survives contact with the enemy. Just last week I spent the best part of a day trying to re-boot a crashed computer. We have to accept that things will always happen to throw our schedules out of synch. That's life, don't stress it!

The second method is to make a list of all the things you have to do that day. This is the method my wife uses. We have a large chalkboard in the kitchen on which she lists all the current chores and jobs. You can list them in order of priority, and then assign a specific time to each. This could be as simple as *Wash the car - Wednesday. Fix the gate - Thursday,*

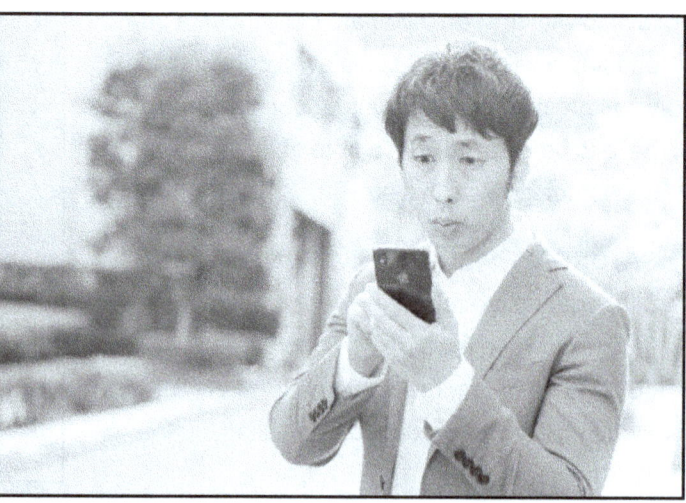

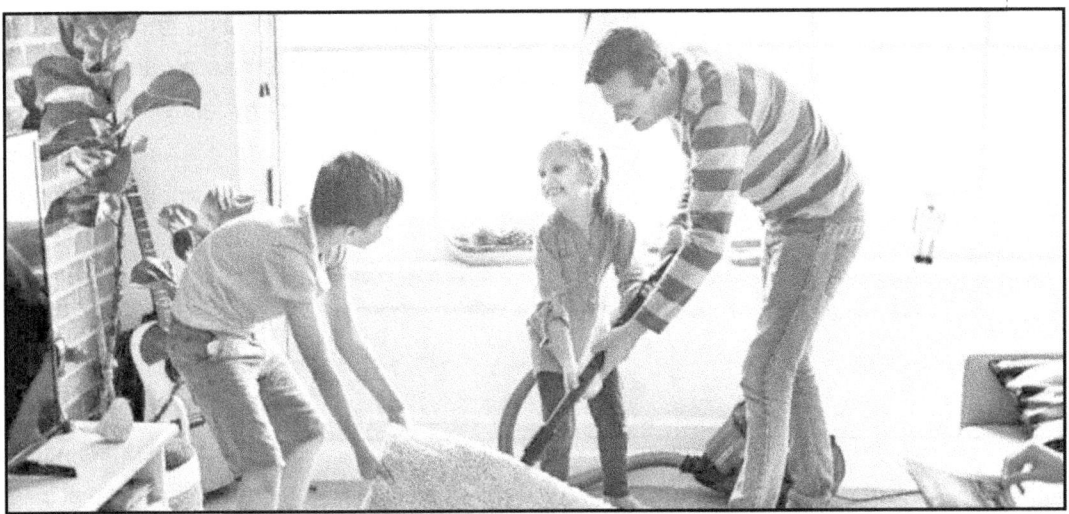

or it may be a detailed daily timetable.

Of course, you will probably end up blending the two methods together in some way. The important thing is that you are taking control and ownership of how you spend your time. Failure to do this means we are either bobbing about, at the mercy of whichever particular wave happens to come our way (reacting to events rather than responding to them), or we suddenly find we are spending five hours a day on the X-box while the house falls down around our ears!

Both of these methods require a little forethought and planning ahead, which is no bad thing. Factor this into your schedule - you could perhaps set aside thirty minutes each Sunday evening in order to draw up a rough schedule for the week ahead. This could be quite vague, just assigning various task to various days. You could then spend ten minutes at the start of each day to draw up a more detailed routine. Once you get the hang of it, it doesn't take long. And, of course, you will start to establish patterns that work best for you.

Be realistic with your timings and try to keep things in balance. Remember, this is not about never giving yourself any time off it's about giving a little shape to your life, establishing some balanced routines. Don't get too hung up on keeping everything perfect and running like a well-oiled machine - our aim is to decrease stress, not increase it!

Also, don't think you have to schedule every minute of your day - it's fine to have an hour or so put aside where nothing is due to happen! This will also help give you a bit more time if something unexpected crops up, or gives you a space you can fill with a relaxing activity. In any case, be sure to schedule in

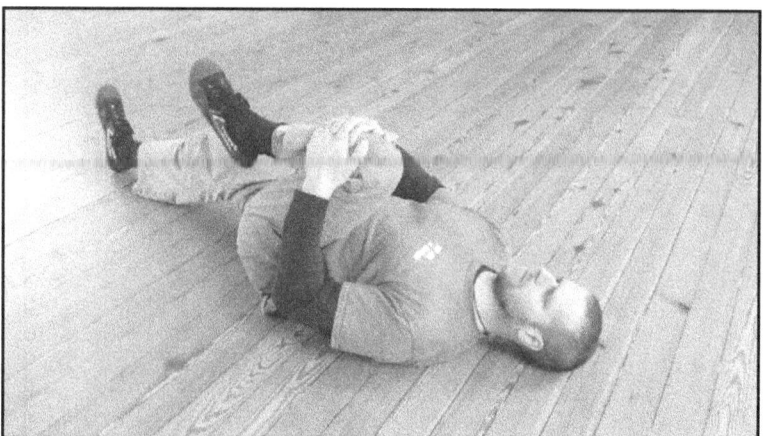

breaks too! As I mentioned before, for every hour you spend on a computer, or sat at a disk, put in five minutes activity. It might be just walking around, having a bit of a stretch, or popping outside for some fresh air. Anything to change your posture and get you away from staring at a screen.

I'll mention exercise routines here, too. Generally speaking the mainstream approach to exercise is that we set aside some time each day for our workout. We go to the gym at a set time, or we get on the exercise bike when we get home from work. That's fine but there are other ways to approach how we exercise.

My own preference is to view exercise as activity rather than chore. These days, I rarely set aside a daily slot specifically for exercise. Instead, I build my training into my other activities. Taking the dogs for a run means I can work my Ladder Breathing. Waiting for the kettle to boil - squats and press ups. Sitting at a desk - shoulder rotations and selective tension.

This also means that my exercise relates specifically to my activities - in other words, it is functional fitness. I find this approach keeps my exercise fresh and so don't get stuck into the same old "numbers" routines, which can get a bit like being on a treadmill - it is mindless activity rather than mindful. The downside is you need to be self disciplined to do this but you could always add it into your written schedule!

Having dependents is another way to establish routines. It may be children, it may be pets or livestock. Either way, they all need to be fed, watered and cleaned up after! That leads us on to the question of demands on our time and how we respond to them. Some demands are non-negotiable - feeding a baby, for example. Though even in that situation, it is always okay to ask for help. At other times, we must have the ability to say no.

LEARNING TO SAY NO

Did you ever encounter one of those people who likes you to do everything for them? I had that experience a couple of years back with a work colleague. It started out reasonably enough, could I help with this, would I mind doing that? But after a period of a few months, I suddenly realised that I was doing almost all of this person's publicity and on-line work, and was expected to be doing even more. He was even messaging me to do things while I was away on holiday! I had to make a decision, and that decision was to start saying *no!*

Now, you don't have to be so blunt and direct - though sometimes that may be called for. My own approach was to start saying "I won't be able to do that right now, perhaps in a week or so," or to say "No, I'm too busy to take on anything else at the moment." Before that, I'd even tried offering to teach the person how to do his own online work, though he showed little interest in that.

The demanding person may be a work colleague, it may be a family member of friend. What they ask you to do may appear quite trivial. "Make me a cup of tea, would you?" or it may end up taking over your life and causing considerable stress. Frequently, this kind of behaviour starts out quite small and grows. In more extreme cases it is a form of grooming, leading to one person's life being almost totally controlled by a partner.

The first step is to recognise that this is something that is happening in your life. Are you the person who always ends up clearing up? Are you the one who always drives? Does your neighbour have half of your DIY and gardening tools and never gives them back? Does your boss or colleague keep asking you to work late to help out, or giving you extra work? This sort of thing can not only play havoc with your time management - in effect, you are at someone else's beck and call. It can also create resentment, which leads to stress, Double stress, in fact, as you feel not only put-upon but are also unable to do the other things that you wanted to do.

In a work environment, there may be procedures in place that you can turn to. Are you able to talk to a manager, trade union rep or personnel officer about the situation? Will speaking directly to the person involved and telling them how you feel help?

In a relationship, it can be a little more difficult. That may be visiting people that you don't really

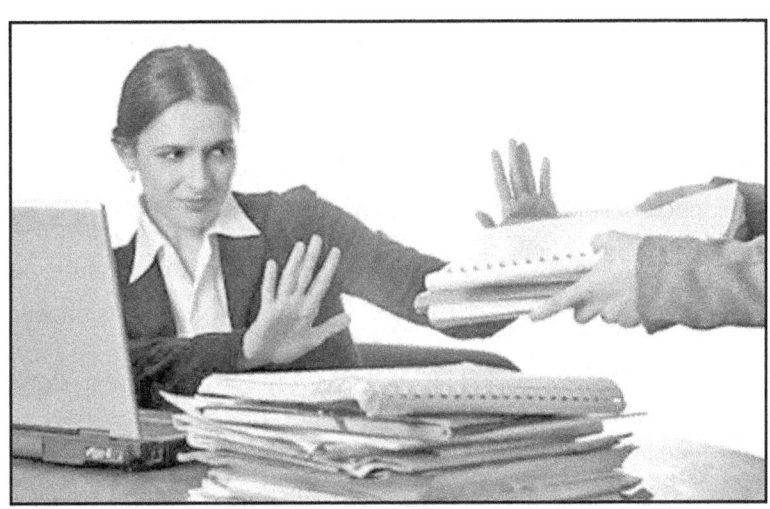

like, it may be getting involved in activities you don't enjoy or are not comfortable with. While there are compromises in all relationships, there are also "lines in the sand", so to speak. Is your partner aware of your feelings? Explaining them may help. If not, it may be that there are deeper issues that need to be addressed in the relationship.

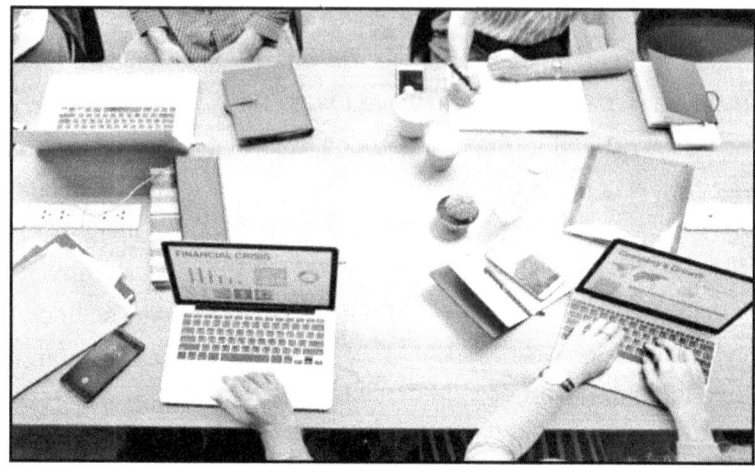

Sometimes we think that saying no makes us a bad person, rude, or selfish. This is another of those unhelpful beliefs, though it may be useful to trace where they come from. Quite often they stem from childhood - we were taught that saying "no" was not polite. You may even have even been scolded for refusing to do something. As adults, we are capable of making our own choices, as well as knowing the difference between right and wrong. Therefore, *no* shouldn't be a forbidden word, but something that we decide on ourselves, based on our own discretion. However, we often hold onto our childhood beliefs and continue to associate *no* with being bad mannered, unkind, or selfish. If we say no, we may feel guilty, or ashamed

Another aspect of learning to say no is realizing that you are valuable and that your time and opinion are as important as anyone else's. If you live your life always depending on other people's approval, you will never feel happy. We must each learn to value ourselves as individuals, accepting that we occasionally make mistakes, but not allowing those mistakes to define us. No one has the right to bully, cajole or manipulate us into doing things we do not wish to do.

The third aspect to learning to say no is deciding if saying yes is really worth it. Have you ever accepted an invitation to an event you didn't really want to go to? You then spend the next two weeks thinking up a good excuse to tell your hosts! Isn't it easier to politely decline in the first place?

The question, then, is how do we best say *no*? Of course it depends largely on the circumstances, but here are a few tips:

Be direct. Don't say *perhaps* or *maybe*.

Don't apologize and give a long list of reasons.

Don't lie. Lying will most likely lead to stress,

and this is what we are trying to avoid.

Be polite, such as saying *thanks for asking.*

Practice saying no. Imagine a scenario and then practice saying no either by yourself or with a friend. This will get you feeling a lot more comfortable with saying no.

Don't say *I'll think about it* if you don't want to do it. This will just prolong the situation and make you feel even more stressed.

Above all, remember that your self-worth does not depend on how much you do for other people.

Learning to say no can help us to feel we have control over our lives and can free us from feeling trapped, resentful, or guilty. These feelings also relate to how positive or negative our outlook is, which forms part of our thinking habits.

POSITIVE THINKING

You might think that saying "no" indicates negative thinking, and that can certainly be the case. The trick is to use saying no in a positive way and not to make it your standard response. Winston Churchill once said: "A pessimist sees the difficulty in every opportunity. An optimist sees the opportunity in every difficulty."

I'm sure we all know people who see the worse in every situation. My wife describes this type of person as *always has a reason not to do something.* It can be an easy mindset fall into and I can't help thinking that such a negative outlook becomes a self-fulfilling prophecy. If nothing else, people will eventually stop inviting such a miserable so-and-so to do anything!

How can we turn a negative mindset around? One way is to literally "count our blessings." You can add this in to your journal, or keep a separate account. Basically, note down each time something nice happens to you. It can be the smallest thing, perhaps someone gave you a cheery *Morning!* on the way to work. Alternatively, last thing at night, before you go to sleep, spend a few minutes running through all the good things that happened to you that day. Bear in mind also, that positivity is contagious and that what goes round, comes round, as the saying goes. Try committing a random act of kindness during the day. Again, these don't have

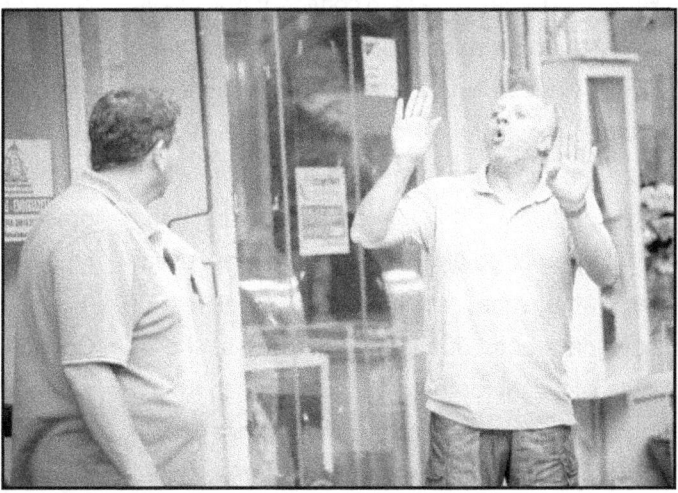

to be huge displays of generosity, simply paying for someone's coffee will bring a smile. They don't even have to be overt, you could put some money in a charity tin, or donate to a food bank.

If we are constantly suffering from negative thoughts, how can we counter them? One approach is to try and analyse the situation from an outside perspective. Take your feelings out of the picture and think about things logically. Over the years, I've been for countless auditions as a musician. I've also been involved in session work, which usually means turning up to a studio to record parts for people you've never met before. In both cases, you are putting yourself on the line. There has not been one occasion where, on the drive there, I haven't thought, *"Am I really up to this? I could give them a call, tell them I can't make it. I could be back home in ten minutes."*

And every single time I have ignored that voice. How? Partly because I am confident that I have a reasonable standard of ability in my playing. I'm no virtuoso but have enough experience to handle most things thrown at me. Partly because subscribe to the view *what's the worst that can happen?"* In this case, the worst thing would be not getting the job. That may be for several reasons - ability is only one aspect of being in a band, it might be that my sound or style isn't right for the group. Perhaps there's a logistical issue, perhaps they have other people to see. Sometimes personalities clash, we can't get on with everyone and we have to recognise that. So, preparation and willingness to accept "failure" are some ways to counter negativity. With those comes a level of confidence and, once again, confidence is contagious.

Imagine you are listening to a presentation by two different speakers. The first walks hesitantly to the podium, drops his notes, can't find his glasses, coughs and stammers his way into his speech.

The second speaker strides up, has no notes, fixes the audience with a smile and begins. Which would you consider the greater expert? Of course, this may all be sham - confidence is no guarantee of ability. There are people, such as politicians, who are trained in oratory and similar skills, regardless of how much they actually know about the topic at hand.

Generally, though, people respond well to a confident approach, it reassures them. This is not to say you should present a false front, or that you should always take the lead of the loudest person in the group. Confidence is not necessarily noisy! Just think about how you present yourself, how you come across in this type of situation.

Confidence thrives on preparation, so if the potentially stressful event is a known quantity, do your best to prepare for it. That may be something specific - a job interview, a speech.

It may be something more general - having to deal with members of the public or an overbearing boss. In these cases, there are preparations that can be made, be it reading up on your subject or even getting some training in public speaking or assertiveness.

Re-framing the experience is another way to over-come negativity. We learn to always look for the silver lining or, as we mentioned in the earlier chapter, learn to place things in context. There is a famous Chinese proverb that illustrates this perfectly:

A farmer had only one horse. One day, his horse ran away. His neighbours said, "I'm so sorry. This is such bad news. You must be so upset."

The man just said, "We'll see."

A few days later, his horse came back with twenty wild horses following. The man and his son corralled all 21 horses. His neighbours said, "Congratulations! This is such good news. You must be so happy!"

The man just said, "We'll see."

A short while later, one of the wild horses kicked the man's only son, breaking both his legs. His neighbours said, "I'm so sorry. This is such bad news. You must be so upset."

The man just said, "We'll see."

The country went to war, and every able-bodied young man was drafted to fight. The war was terrible and killed every young man, but the farmer's son was spared, since his broken legs prevented him from being drafted. His neighbours said, "Congratulations! This is such good news. You must be so happy!"

The man just said, "We'll see."

The moral of the story is that what sometimes seems like a negative event may turn out to have a positive side. We don't always recognise what is a blessing and what is a curse. It also points to the fact that negative experiences can be temporary and shot-lived.

Keep an eye, then, on your thinking habits. Note if you tend to be overly negative or pessimistic, if you have low self-esteem or are over-critical.

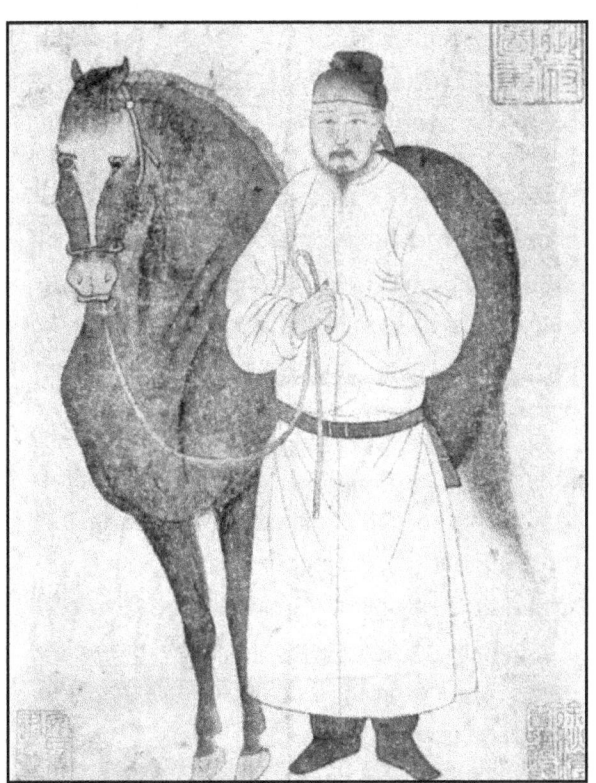

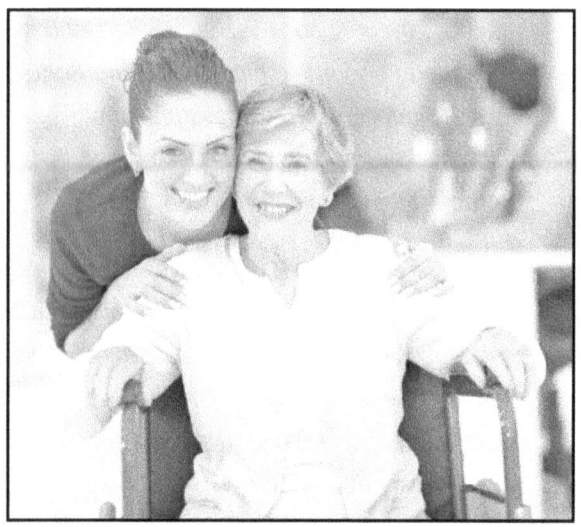

SLEEP

How much sleep do you think you need? The answer varies according to age but for most adults, the general recognised ideal amount is 7-9 hours per night. Young children tend to need more, the elderly a little less. The amount may also vary according to different conditions - pregnancy, for example. However, for most of use, we are looking at an average of eight hours sleep per night. But sleep is just one aspect of a natural cycle, or what is called our Circadian Rhythm

Also take care not to think in absolutes, not to over-indulge in wishful thinking, and to balance ambitions with ability and reality. Be tolerant of others and their faults but also be aware of people who take advantage. Don't get too fixed, be open to new ways of thinking and doing things.

One last piece of advice on mindset, and that is simply to smile! Researchers at the University of Kansas published research showing that smiling actually helps reduce the body's response to stress. Many other studies link smiling to lower blood pressure, and even to longevity.

Even faking a smile may be beneficial! It seems that doing so does not reduce stress in the moment, but speeds recovery when a stressful experience is over. Smiling can also be contagious, in fact there are some therapies based around group laughing. *Smile and the world smiles with you!*

CIRCADIAN RHYTHM

Have you ever noticed that you feel either energised or drowsy around the same times every day? This is down to your circadian rhythm, a 24-hour internal clock that is runs in the background of your brain and cycles between sleepiness and alertness at regular intervals. It's also known as your sleep/wake cycle.

For most adults, the biggest dips in energy occur between 2am and 4am, and around 1pm to 3pm. If you are getting good, regular sleep, you won't notice these dips so much. However, if you have a poor sleep pattern, you'll notice bigger swings of sleepiness and alertness.

Our circadian rhythm is largely controlled by the hypothalamus, though outside factors such as darkness and light can also have an influence. For example, at night, our eyes send a signal to the hypothalamus that it's time to feel tired. The brain then sends a signal to your body to release melatonin, which makes the body tired. That's why circadian rhythms tend to coincide with the cycle of daytime and nighttime and why it can be hard hard for shift workers to sleep during the day and remain awake at night.

Circadian rhythm works best when we have regular sleep habits. Any change to that routine - jet lag, staying up late and so on - may have an effect. Needless to say, stress can also disrupt our natural rhythms. This is a double-effect as our circadian clock also plays a big part in regulating the immune system and any disruption to that will also have a negative impact on our metabolism.

STAGES OF SLEEP

As we discussed before, our brain states change in the various stages of sleep. The stages are:

Light - the brain waves slow, body temperature drops. This normally lasts for around half an hour.

Deep - heart rate and breathing slow, blood pressure drops. Our system goes into restorative mode, initiating tissue repair and regeneration. Usually lasts for around 90 minutes.

REM (Rapid Eye Movement) - our deepest stage, where we dream. Very important for psychological health. Also higher levels of growth hormone are produced. REM is around ten minutes long at first, growing longer, up to an hour.

Throughout the night, we cycle between these three stages, with REM taking up about 25% of the time.

INSOMNIA

Insomnia is the technical term for difficulty in sleeping. We all suffer from it to some degree at various times in our lives and it can become a chronic condition. The most common form of insomnia is known as psycho-physiological insomnia. This is not related to any physical or mental health issue, but is based purely around the interaction between our thoughts and feelings and our body systems. In other words, what is going on in our minds is forcing the body to stay awake.

Stress is obviously a major trigger factor here. I'm sure we've all had a sleepless night worrying about the bills, or anticipating a big event. Our thoughts set off the adrenal response and, before we know it, the heart is racing, our legs are twitching, the mind is out of control.

COUNTERING INSOMNIA

There are two approaches to getting a good night's sleep. The first is the immediate

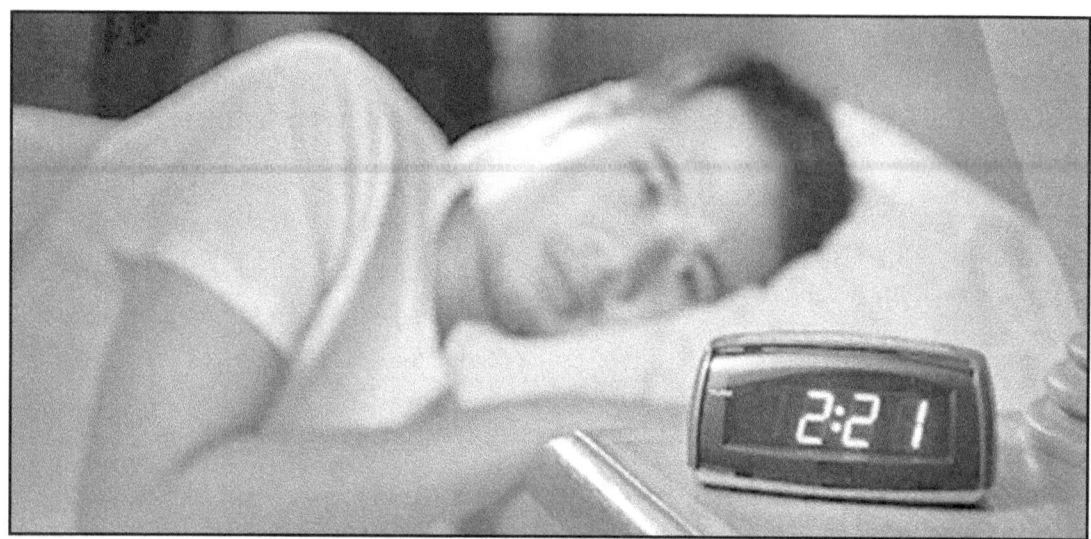

response to the situation. In other words we are in bed and cannot sleep. For this we refer back to our earlier breathing exercises - Quiet Sitting, Selective Tension, and so on. These should go a long way into damping down our adrenal response and so allow body and mind to relax.

Counting sheep sounds like such a cliche but it, or something similar, can work very well. Concentrating on a mundane but slightly detailed task distracts the mind away from the cause of the worry. Sometimes it is best to get up and be active for a short time. We know that movement helps dissipate the adrenal dump, so do some light stretching or similar. Avoid activities that stimulate the brain too much - don't check your phone, for example. Personally, reading always works for me. A few pages and I'm usually drifting off again.

In some circumstances, you might want to look at taking sleeping tablets. There are various types available, the herbal varieties appeal more to me than other types. I would recommend this only on rare occasions, as it's not something you want to make a habit of.

The second approach is to be pre-emptive and think about what we are doing before we go to bed. Probably the most constructive change we can make is to avoid electronics before bedtime. That means TV's, computers, mobile phones. Looking at any of these late at night exposes the brain to blue light, which tells your brain that it's light out, so it needs to be awake. Some claim that effect can last for up to two hours!

Keep an eye on what you eat and sleep before bedtime. Caffeine is an obvious no-no but nicotine and sugar are also stimulants. It's best not to eat a heavy meal a few hours before going to bed, particularly spicy foods. People may think that alcohol or other substances will help them sleep. Research, however, has shown that students who drank before bed had interrupted sleep patterns. Alcohol may reduce the time it takes to get to sleep but it causes wakefulness in the second half of the night, counteracting the benefit. Anyone who's been up and down three times a night to the loo can confirm that!

There are activities that will help us to sleep. A relaxing bath before bed, reading, Quiet Sitting, a warm, milky drink. Our environment is obviously also important. I once live in a house that had a street light right outside the front bedroom window. We ended up having to buy very heavy drapes to block out the light as it was affecting our sleep.

Noise is another factor and one that may be out of our control. A neighbour's dog that barks all night, music, alarms going off. If these are regular occurrences, address them as best you can. An alternative would be to try earplugs or an eye mask. It is often worth having these in your bag if you travel a lot. On occasion I've had to stay in a hotel that had a disco downstairs that goes on til early morning - not ideal!

Think also about the bed itself. Perhaps a new mattress would help, are the pillows comfortable? Is the temperature right in the room - too hot can be as bad as too cold.

You should also take into account your personal rhythms and lifestyle. Some of us are early birds, some of us are night owls - personally, I'm much better late at night than first thing in the morning! Work and social activities will largely determine when you can sleep, so look at both of those areas to see if there is room for change.

TAKING NAPS

Having an occasional nap is a good way to boost energy levels. The Japanese call this *Inemuri,* which translates as "sleeping while present." A good nap can bring almost as many benefits as a full night's sleep. Some schools of thought suggest that we should always sleep naturally, as animals do - ie, when we are tired. Obviously this is not practical for most of us, particularly if you are a bus driver! And, as we have already

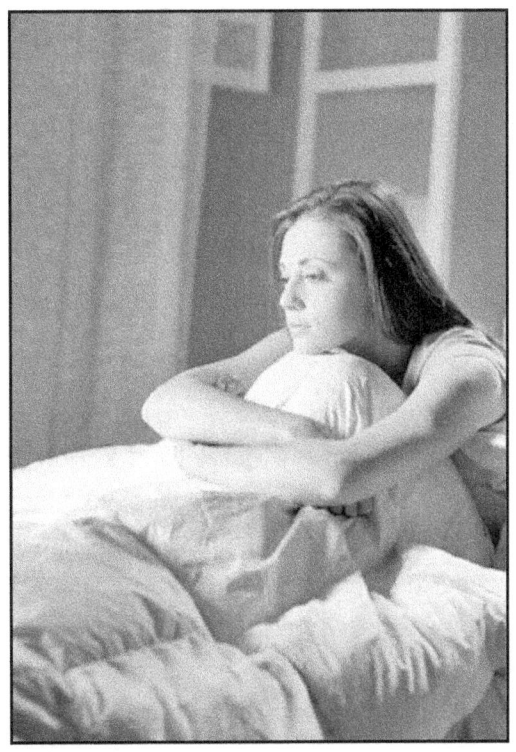

noted, we should naturally feel more tired at night time. However, if you do feel very tired and it is not inappropriate to do so, having a nap can work wonders. Countries that have *siestas* understand this well!

The key to napping is doing it at the right time. Napping too late can prevent you from sleeping at night, and napping for too long can cause grogginess (called *sleep inertia*). If you go to bed quite late (midnight), the best time to nap is around 2:30 - 3 pm. If you go to bed earlier, the best time to nap is around 1 - 1:30 pm.

THE POWER NAP

This takes 15-20 minutes, and is long enough to get the benefits of a nap without getting too groggy, as you wake before the brain enters deep sleep. This type of nap has been shown to boost your energy, alertness and learning ability. It's also a good way to make up for sleep deficit from a poor night's sleep. Longer naps are possible but they will take us into the deeper sleep states. That means taking longer to "wake-up" afterwards.

Find a comfortable place where you will not be disturbed, loosen any tight clothing, kick off your shoes. The easiest way to control your length of nap is to set an alarm. Add an extra five minutes on to give yourself time to nod off. When you wake up, you can expose yourself to sunlight and do some exercise to ensure your circadian rhythms are not disturbed.

DIET

Hardly a month goes by without a new diet coming onto the market. It's actually nothing new, diets have been around for centuries and have ranged from the sensible to the ridiculous (the cotton ball diet is actually a real thing!). I'm not going to present any specific diets here, as they very much depend on individual circumstances. We will take a look, though, at diet as it relates to stress and tension.

We all know that what we eat has a major effect on our health and well-being. So the first thing we should ensure is that we are getting a balanced diet.

BALANCED DIET

A balanced diet is one that provides the body with all the essential nutrients, vitamins and minerals it needs to maintain cells, tissues and organs as well as to function correctly. A diet lacking in nutrients can lead to health problems that range from lack of energy to serious problems with the function of vital organs. A balanced diet includes foods from all the healthy food groups in the correct proportions. It should also be made up of the correct number of calories in order for us to maintain a healthy weight, and ideally be low in processed foods.

As each of us is different, correct diet will change from person to person. However, following a diet that is varied, covers all food groups and is low

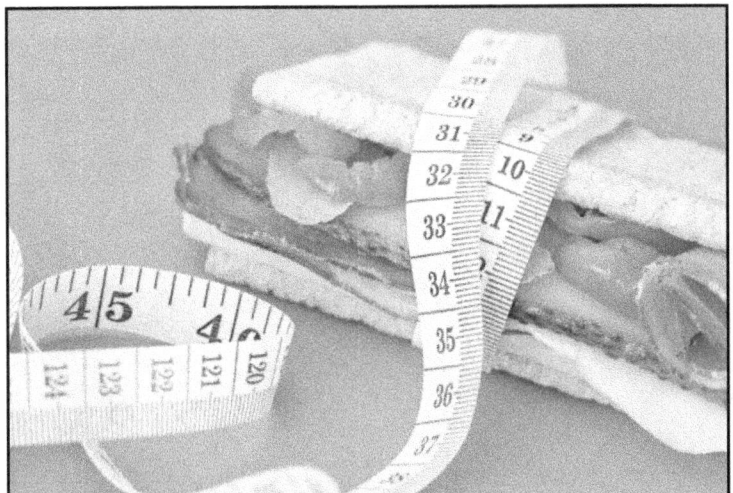

in undesirables such as sugar, is a good start to maintaining health. Ideally, we should be eating at least three meals a day. Each meal should include something from each food group and portion sizes should be moderated to control calorie intake. That calorie intake should also be balanced with physical activity. To cut it down to its most basic, take Billy Connolly's advice: "if you want to lose weight, eat less and move around more!"

Limiting alcohol consumption is also recommended. Current UK guidelines are that we drink a maximum of 14 units per week (one unit is equal to half a pint of beer or a small glass of wine.) Drink free days are also recommended.

The Food Groups are:

1. Dairy - cheese, milk and yoghurt. Usually high in saturated fats, so choose low fat or fat free varieties. Dairy is essential for calcium for strong bones, protein and vit D. Possible replacements include soy or nut based milks.

2. Protein - lean meat, poultry, fish, legumes, nuts, eggs and soy proteins such as tofu. Meat and poultry are high in iron, whilst legumes are a rich source of fibre. Eggs also provide a multitude of vitamins and minerals. Oily fish is high in omega three fatty acids.

Cooking methods should be low fat - grilling, poaching, dry frying or steaming. Be aware that processed meats, such as sausages, may be high in fat and sodium.

3. Fruit - virtually fat free, low in calories, high in fibre and nutritious. Include a variety in your diet to get a wide range of vitamins and minerals. Be careful with fruit juices, they often contain extra sugar.

4. Vegetables - generally contain the least calories and the most vitamins and minerals. Again, include a variety in your meals to get different vitamins. Best cooking methods are steaming or grilling.

5. Grains - our major carbohydrate source, includes bread, cereals, pasta and rice. Try to choose whole-grain varieties as these are higher in fibre and contain more B vitamins. Avoid sugary breakfast cereals and sweetened

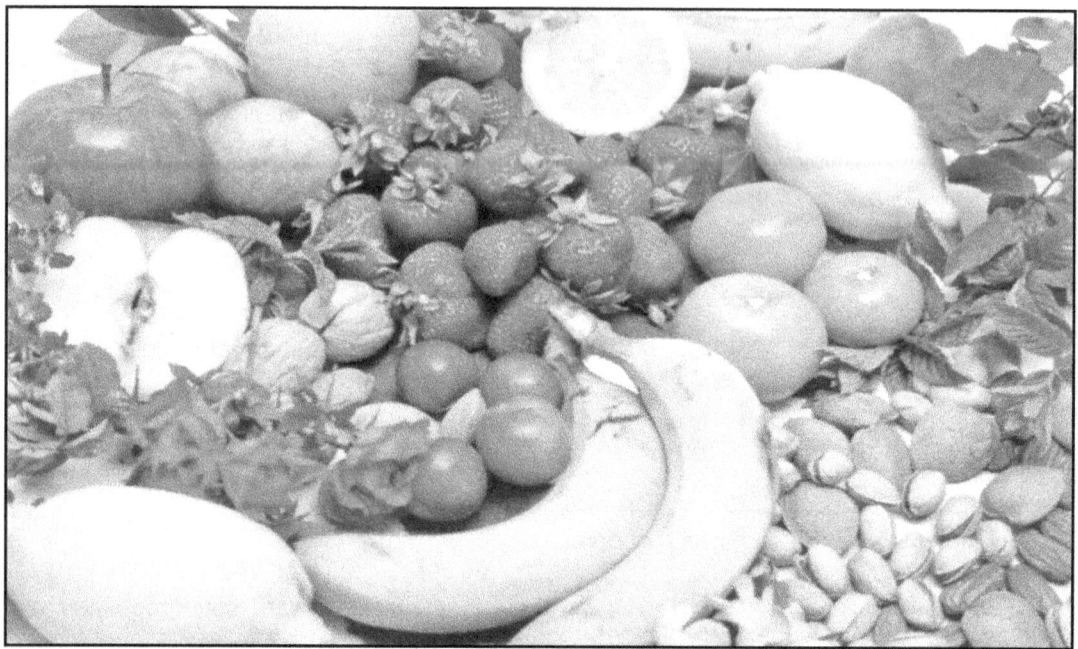

breads made with refined flour as these contain little fibre and are higher in calories and fat.

6. Fats and Oils - fat is necessary in our diets but it is important to choose the right types. Saturated and trans fats should be minimized, or replaced with vegetable fats such as olive or sunflower oil or spreads. All fats contain a high amount of calories, so it is important to keep added fats to a minimum. Other good sources of unsaturated fats include nuts, avocado and fish.

7. Treats - foods that do not fit into the above groups are generally considered to provide little nutritional benefit and are therefore not required in a balanced diet. That includes sweets, chocolate, cakes, crisps and so on. If you do indulge in a treat, try to minimise calorie intake.

STRESS-RELATED EATING

There are two conditions related to stress and food. The first is *comfort eating*, where we treat ourselves or binge on, usually, unhealthy foods to relieve our stress. The second is not eating enough, as we are "too busy" to cook, or living on a diet of junk food. We may also substitute things for food - cigarettes or alcohol being the prime contenders. Either of these may develop into more serious conditions, such as bulimia, which require specialised treatment.

Again, we all have off-days and, as I've said before there's nothing wrong every now and then with watching a weepy film and ploughing through a box of chocolates. But if this is happening every week, there is obviously an issue.

You should also not think of a diet as a "punishment." Much like our exercise, think of eating as an enjoyable activity rather than something you have to endure. With a little thought and seasoning you can make even the most bland food more tasty. So let's look at some guidelines for both monitoring our diet and also how we eat.

Set aside time for meals - it's quite common to see, in TV advertising especially, the "successful" person who is on the go 24-7. They flow from work (eating at the desk) to nightclub (with no dinner) before grabbing the guy/girl and going home. They somehow manage to look fantastic the whole time, too! Fantastic is the word, it's pure fantasy.

I remember seeing an ad break when I was in the US a few years back. The "too busy to eat, so grab one of our highly processed snacks" ads was followed by an ad for heartburn relief!

So, as much as you can, once a day if practical, set aside a meal time. It might be breakfast, lunch or dinner. Turn off your phone and TV. Prepare a nice, balanced meal, then sit at a table and eat it slowly. Be aware of your food - its colour, texture, smell and taste. Savour each mouthful. When you are finished, sit for a few minutes to let your food "go down."

Avoid comfort eating - when you have a stress trigger, be aware if you find yourself reaching for food. In my case it's always chocolate! That big bar that usually lasts for a couple of days might disappear in one go! Here, we are using food to calm the mind. Instead, try some of our other remedies, such as breathing, movement, etc. If you absolutely have to have something to eat, go for a healthy option, such as nuts.

Hunger check - before you eat, check if your hunger is physical or emotional. Are you eating because you are bored? Monitor your meal

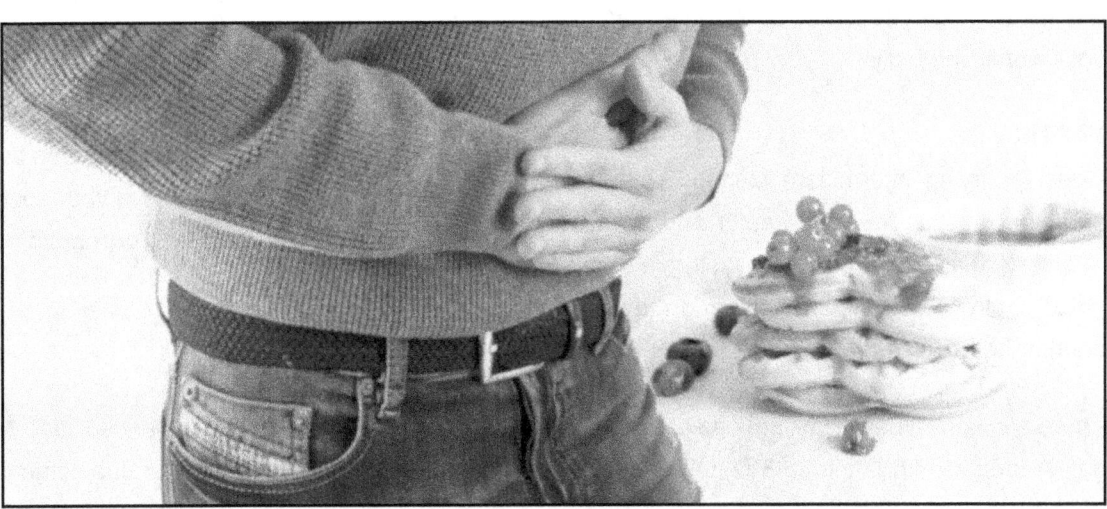

portions. Stop eating when you are full. If you have a lot of food left on the plate, make smaller portions. Of course, diet is something you can easily add into your journal. This is also a good way of monitoring exactly what we are eating and how it makes us feel. Try varying your diet to see what works best for you.

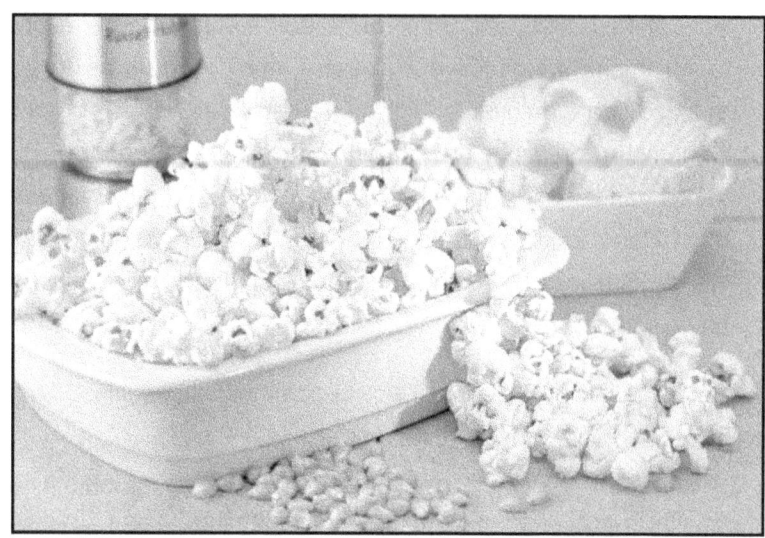

Be aware of intolerance or allergies - a while back I found I was feeling constantly bloated. Even after a light meal, my stomach would feel full and tight. Eventually, I had some tests and discovered I was wheat intolerant. Now, by watching my food intake, I've largely got rid of the bloating. It may be gluten, grains or dairy, so if you are having problems ask your doctor to check for you. Another way is to keep a food diary and cut out certain foods. Monitor any changes in your condition and adjust your diet accordingly.

FASTING

Consider trying intermittent fasting. This is a common practice in many health and spiritual traditions. It gives our digestive system a break, helps control blood sugar levels and may help counter heart disease.

There are many types of fasting. The easiest and safest to start with is the 16:8 fast. This simply means that for 16 hours of each day you consume nothing but unsweetened beverages like water, coffee, and tea. You eat all your meals and snacks in the remaining eight hours.

If you include sleep in your fasting hours, then we are really only not eating for eight hours a day. So you might restrict eating to between the hours of 11 am and 7pm. Remember, at this stage you are taking in liquids during your fast period.

More advanced methods call for 24 hours with no food or water, but this is something to be built up to, if required. Always check with your doctor first and be sure to monitor your condition throughout.

VITAMINS & SUPPLEMENTS

If you are eating a healthy, balanced diet you should have little or no need for supplements.

However, there may be times when our diet or circumstances change. As far as stress goes, it is the B vitamins that may help us the most, by boosting brain chemistry and function. Research by Swinburne University, Australia, in 2014 revealed that chronic stress depletes levels of vitamin B6 in the body. The study also showed a 20% reduction in work-related stress in those consuming higher levels of B vitamins.

A 2004 study published in the British Medical Journal found that folate can help improve mood, while a 2013 review by Swansea University confirmed that high doses of B vitamins may be effective in improving mood states. Unlike many other vitamins, B vitamins are not stored in the body, they are water-soluble, so get flushed out within hours if they're not used. A good diet should give us all the B vitamins we need but you may want to consider topping up your daily levels at stressful times.

There's a huge range of supplements available, from herbal remedies to minerals to roots. With such a wide variety available and so many claims made, it can be difficult to determine which, if any, supplements you need and which will work. I can only suggest you do as much research as possible and try not to take too much notice of advertising blurb. It is always a good idea to speak to your doctor or other professional too.

WORK LIFE BALANCE`

The final lifestyle strategy we will look at is achieving balance in our lives. This is usually defined as work-life balance but the principles apply to any of our activities. We should aim to achieve equilibrium in our relationships, in our hobbies, in all our dealings with others.

Finding the right balance between life and work isn't just about the number of hours you devote to one or the other. It's about establishing a set of priorities and committing the time you have outside of work towards improving what's important to you. That balance will inevitably shift at times, as circumstances change but having a set of clearly defined goals, rather than

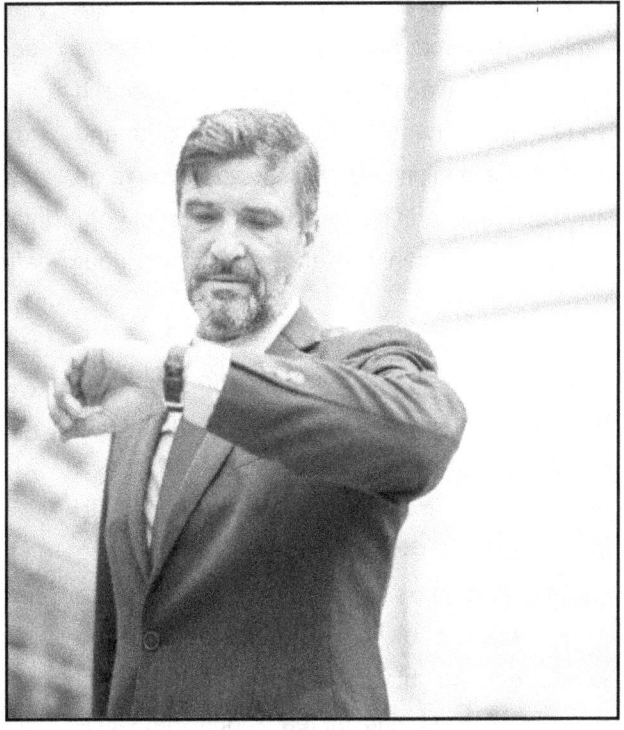

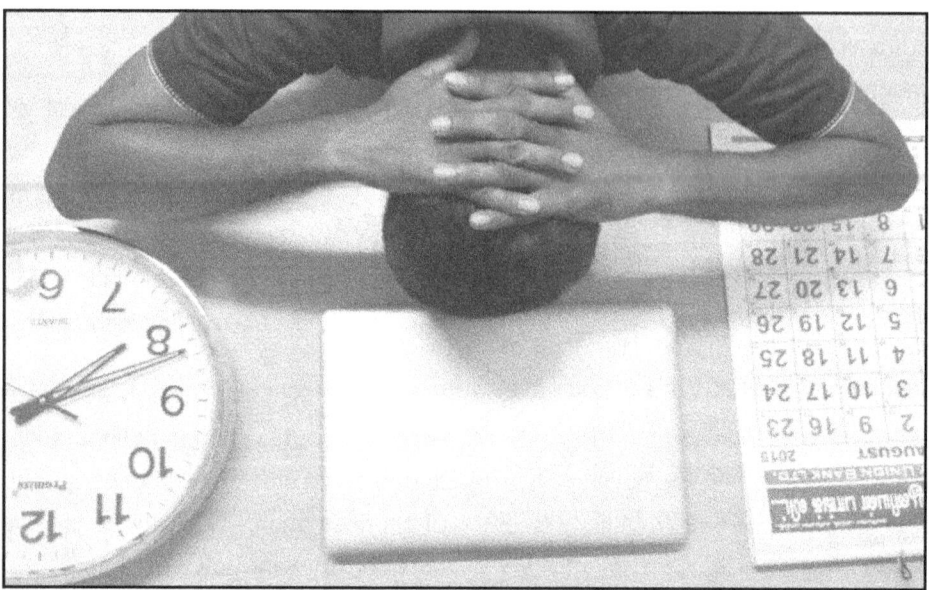

rigid schedules, we can soon achieve a balanced and flexible lifestyle.

The first step to achieving this is to break the cycle of overwork and overstress. That means learning to leave your work at the workplace. If you habitually bring your work home, or spend a lot of time thinking about work when you're off the clock, then adding variety to the rest of your life will help to minimise the prominence your job.

Also consider the effort you put into your work and seriously evaluate what you're getting back out of it. While it might be reasonable to work a fifty hour week for a few months while trying to earn a promotion, working those hours non-stop for little in return is not. You may wish to strive for perfection or always go above and beyond what's required but without any pay-off, the cost is your own well-being. Instead, apply that same determination to areas of your life that will make you happier and more fulfilled.

The second thing to do is set yourself a schedule - particularly when it comes to electronic devices. It can be almost impossible to detach from work with notifications coming in via e-mail, text, etc round the clock. Give yourself a deadline, say eight in the evening, after which you turn your devices off. A 2015 American study showed more than nine out of ten people use devices at or near bedtime. As we have already mentioned, use of these devices interferes with both quality and quantity of sleep.

Next, examine your relationships, determine which are important to you and invest more time in cultivating them. Sometimes we may feel that out relationship obligations outweigh the enjoyment we get from them. It may be that we have negative or even destructive people in our lives. It can be a tough issue to resolve but if possible, reduce the time and influence that those people exert over your life. Turn that into more quality time spent with friends and family, people who you want to be with. Healthy social bonds promote a sense of belonging, acceptance and mental well-being.

The good news is that an increasing number of employers are appreciating the benefits of having happy, productive employees. This has meant an increase in practices such as flexible working hours, after work social and leisure activities, working from home and so on.

If you work for a company that doesn't provide any of these, it may be worth discussing them with your Human Resources department. While you probably won't prompt an immediate change, most employers appreciate feedback and should at least be willing to discuss how they might make improvements.

The other side of work balance is the lack of work. If we are retired or unemployed, how can we best bring some structure to our day? A good way to do this is to build some simple routines into your life - set specific tasks for certain days. Factor in some treats for yourself, too, a visit to a museum, or tea with friends.

Having a good social / family circle is invaluable in these circumstances. If you don't have one, consider taking up a new hobby or joining a group of some kind. . Another possibility is to look at voluntary work or helping out with local charities. This has a double bonus of not only keeping us active but also helping others less fortunate than ourselves.

CHAPTER SEVEN
COPING WITH PAIN AND GRIEF

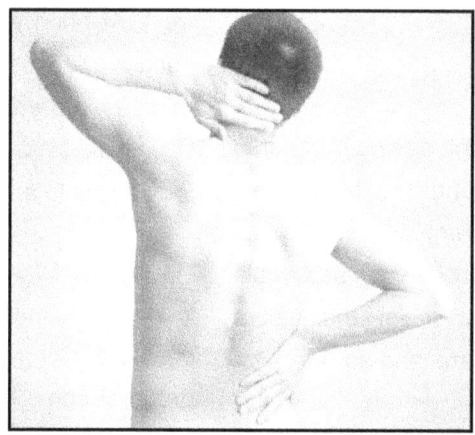

I can't imagine there is a person on the planet who does not experience pain and loss at least once during their lifetime. It may be pain from an injury or illness, it may be the pain of rejection. Loss is usually the result of a bereavement but it could also be the loss of a relationship. Any of these circumstances can bring us pain, be it physical or emotional. But here is the strange thing about pain - it doesn't exist!

What I mean by that is that pain cannot be measured, it cannot be seen, and it is a construct of our imagination. On the other hand, if you've ever had a bad toothache, then you know that pain is very real! So perhaps a better way of talking about pain is to say that it is something we *experience*. Given that, it is easy to understand how different people react to, or even feel pain in very different ways.

Our pain thresholds can change dramatically according to the situation. There are numerous cases of people finishing fights with a broken arm, running a race with a broken leg or of continuing to operate despite being shot. Then again, sometimes a simple knock on the shin has us hopping round the room in agony. Also consider amputees who still feel pain in a missing limb.

The good news from this, is that as pain is largely experienced on a mental level, we should be able to manage it well by accessing and controlling our mental state. In other words, we control our *pain experience*. This is reflected in an old saying, *pain is compulsory, suffering is optional*.

In other words, none of us can avoid pain in life. What we can control is our reaction to it. Let's begin by classifying some different types of pain and how they may impact us.

PHYSICAL PAIN

This type of pain is delivered via our nervous system. It is an indication that there is danger or that something is wrong with the body. Tissues or cells let the nervous system know that they have become inflamed or damaged. The nervous system signals the brain, which evaluates the information in relation to everything else that it is processing. If the brain considers the situation dangerous, it creates a warning signal via the body to correlate with the event, which we then interpret as pain (it could be throbbing, a sharp feeling and so on).

The interesting thing is that there is no "pain centre" in the brain. Instead, the brain draws on memories, emotion, the body map, sense and body systems to create "pain."

This goes some way to explaining how different people react to pain in different ways - we all have different backgrounds, experiences, cultures and so on. It also explains how the memory of pain can feel so real. Either the missing limb example, or when we feel the "twinge" of an old injury, perhaps when in a similar situation to when the injury was first

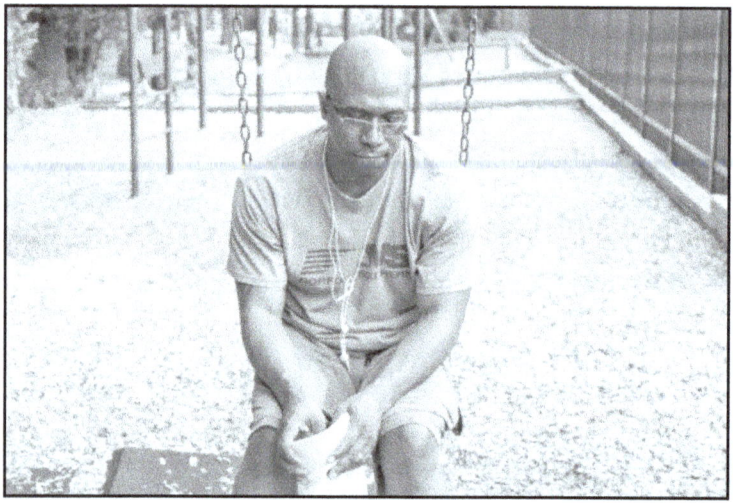

caused. It also explains how the fear of pain can be used to control someone - in an abusive relationship, for example.

To make things even more complicated, that pain experience can further be influenced by our emotional state, how tired we are, if we are adrenalised and so on. Pain can also over-ride itself. Say you have banged your elbow and it hurts. You will likely forget that pain immediately if you then crack your head on the low ceiling beam!

PSYCHOLOGICAL PAIN

This is even more nebulous than physical pain but can be just as debilitating, even leading to self-harm. We have to remember that the mind and body are inextricably linked. Anything that happens in the brain will cause a reaction in our body systems, such as a release of chemicals of hormones or muscular tension. Consequently, we can see that a pained emotional state will also have direct physical consequences. Generally speaking, when sad we feel de-energised, sluggish, weak and tired. Anger or hate tend to take us the other way, we become adrenalised and active.

Again, our experience of pain is down to our memories, our expectations and so on. This time, there is no input from the nervous system as with physical pain. However the physical reaction can be a strong - I've seen people throw up due to shock, or go into an almost comatose state. It is not always immediate, PTSD can manifest long after the actual event. In other cases trauma, whether mental or physical, can become locked into our muscles. We may not even be aware of this, it is as though the body tries to build up an armour in order to protect itself from further hurt.

An interesting thing with emotional pain is how it can be described in a physical way. People talk about feeling *crushed*, for example. Or they experiencing *waves of grief*. An emotional shock may be likened to *a stab in the heart*.

This is important as it also gives us a physical angle form which to approach managing emotional distress, which leads us on to some possible coping strategies.

PAIN CONTROL

There are many different ways to classify pain. For our purposes we will stick to three categories:

Acute pain - also known as sharp pain, something we feel quickly that does not last long. We cut a finger, bang our head on something and so on.

Chronic pain - longer term pain, perhaps caused by a medical condition.

Emotional pain - due to bereavement, relationship issues and so on.

There are some methods that work across all three classifications and the three can also merge into each other. A sharp toothache may be the first sign of a longer term root canal infection which, in turn, will impact our psychological well being. Let's begin at the start though, with that initial, acute pain.

BREATHING

The go to method for sharp pain is to go into Burst Breathing. So, you bang head getting out of the car, think of what your response might be? For some it may be to grab the head with both hands, go into a crouch and go "owww!". This allows the pain to overwhelm us. For a time our entire system is shut down. It is interesting to see how people often "fold" around their pain, or place their hands over it as if trying to hold it in. What we should be doing is throwing the pain away!

So instead of crouching, stand up straight, keep good posture and begin Burst Breathing. Short, sharp breathes, in through the nose, out through the mouth. As you breath, shake your arms and legs. Try not to let any tension that may be creeping into your system take hold. You should find that, after a couple of minutes, the pain has largely gone. As we mentioned before, swearing has also been shown to help relieve short term pain - well, it is a form of Burst Breathing, I suppose!

Just a note - make sure you check for damage. Pain control is not the same as ignoring pain and it is certainly not about "toughing it out." If it needs attention, get it looked at!

Burst Breathing may help in chronic pain for those occasions where the pain becomes

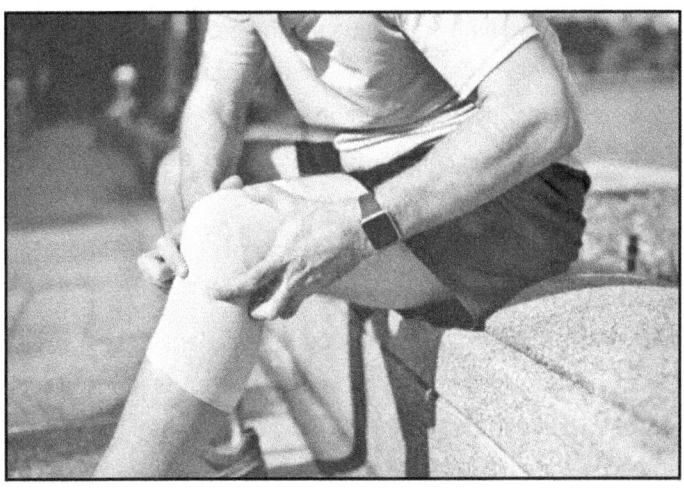

stronger than usual. It may help get you through a rough patch but it is not really designed to be a long term method. For that, we turn to internal awareness.

BODY BRAIN AWARENESS

Body awareness includes the sense of the position and movement of the body (proprioception), the ability to understand the position of one's body and other objects in space (spatial awareness) and a sense of the internal state of the body, cold, hungry, heartbeat, etc (interoception).

Brain awareness means having a good understanding of your emotional self. Understanding your internal process is the first step to being able to control them. Our mental response to any situation is always a choice - we choose to be angry, to be indifferent and so on. Research has shown that people with good mind-body awareness are able to better deal with pain. There are many activities that help develop body awareness, various types of exercises and movement discipline, meditation and so on. Let's first do a simple exercise to give you a basic "body map."

Body Map Exercise

Lay down and run quickly through the Selective Tension exercise from the previous chapter. Get a sense of your muscles, your limbs. Next, feel the size and shape of your body. Get a sense of where your feet are, where you hands are. Feel the weight of your limbs. Compare each side of your body, does the left side feel the same as the right? Now feel the surface of your skin, what are the sensations?

Next, place your awareness in your belly. Try and feel it from the inside. Does it feel empty, or full? Can you feel movement? What are the sensations you feel? Warmth? Pulsing?

After this, place you awareness on your heart. Feel it beating in your chest. Feel how the blood pulses around your body.

Once you can feel this, being to move your extremities. Wiggle your toes and fingers. Slowly start to move your limbs, twist and stretch. Reach across your body - touch the left knee with right hand, for example. When ready, sit up, then stand and return to your normal activities.

Doing this kind of work regularly will give you a good base-view of your body and how it is working. That should make it easier to spot any issues as they arise.

Neuroplasticity

Most types of healthy physical activity will help develop body awareness. Some are specifically designed for this purpose, so taking up one of these will do more than help us physically. Learning new movement skills develops new neural pathways in the brain, what is known as *neuroplasticity*. In short, new physical experiences stimulate our brains into new activities and can also help re-awaken dormant circuitry. This can be of tremendous benefit in certain conditions, such as Parkinsons.

Outside of that, these new pathways better equip us to deal with any type of new information - and we can think of pain as information.

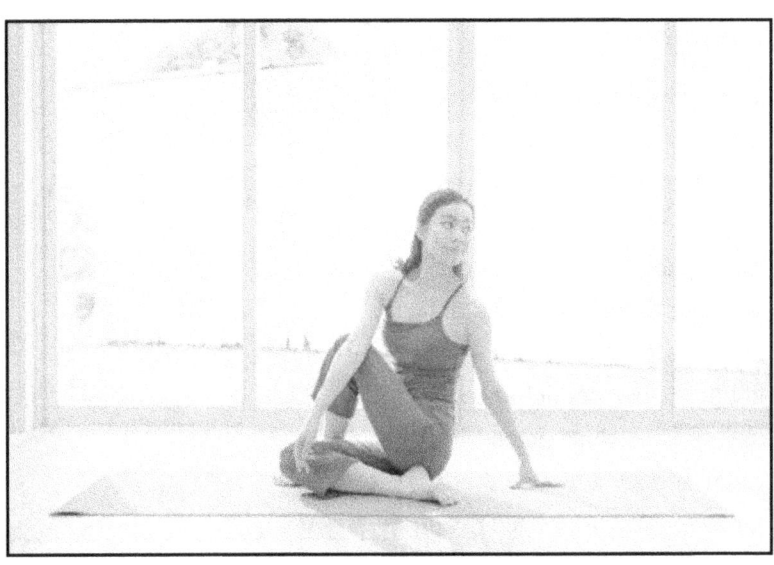

Pain physician and psychiatrist Michael Moskowitz, experienced chronic pain after a series of accidents, so he extensively researched neuroplasticity. He found there are about a dozen regions in the brain where pain is processed, and most of them also do other things. You may have noticed that when you are in pain you get grumpy; that's because one of the areas of the brain that processes pain also processes emotional regulation. Another region processes both pain and the ability to visualise; brain scans show that chronic pain hijacks about 15 per cent of visual processing. Think about how people screw their eyes up when in pain.

Knowing this, Moskowitz's solution was to force himself to visualise whenever he was in pain. The idea was to retake the use of that area of the brain for imagery. After several months practice, he was able to overcome his chronic pain with this method.

MORE VISUALISATION

Let's look at some methods of visualisation to help manage chronic pain. We start with some Quiet Sitting exercises and you need to give yourself a good amount of time for the exercise - maybe thirty minutes or so. You can work in the Selective Tension at the start too, if you wish, to help put yourself in touch with the different parts of your body. When ready, you can try one or more of the following, see which method works best for you.

Altered Focus

Focus your attention on a specific non-painful part of the body and alter the sensation in that part of the body. For example, if the pain is in your shoulder, do not think about it but instead imagine your foot warming up and becoming quite hot. This will take the mind away from focusing on the source of the pain..

Dissociation

This technique involves mentally separating the painful body part from the rest of the body, or imagining the body and mind as separate, with the chronic pain distant from one's mind. For example, imagine your painful knee is sitting on a chair across the room and tell it to stay there, far away from your mind.

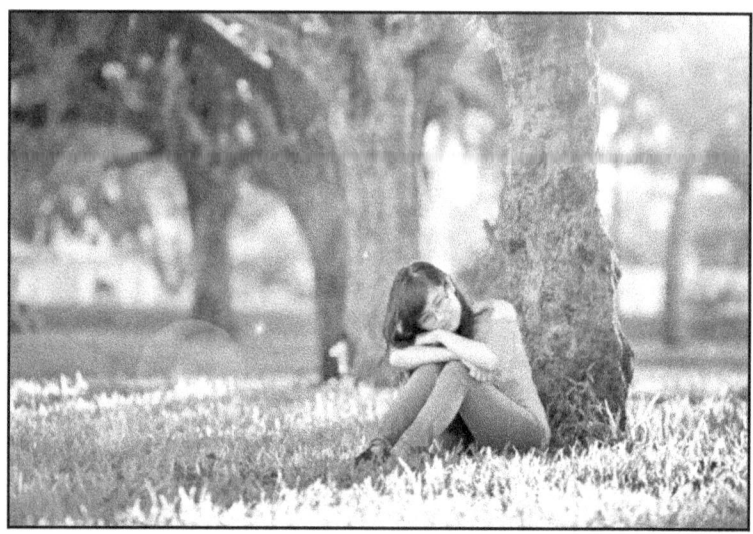

Sensory Splitting

For this method, divide the sensation into separate parts. For example, if the back pain feels hot to you, focus purely on the sensation of heat and not that of the hurting.

Mental Anesthesia

Imagine making an injection of numbing anesthetic into the painful area. Or, you could imagine a soothing heat` pack being placed onto the area of pain. Alternatively, you can imagine your brain producing massive amount of endorphins, the natural pain relieving substance of the body, and having them flow to the painful area of your body.

Transfer

Use your mind to produce altered sensations, such as heat, cold, anesthetic, in a non-painful hand. Next, then place that hand on the painful area and imagine transferring this pleasant sensation from the hand into the pain.

Age Progression/ Regression

Use your mind's eye to project yourself forward or backward in time to when you are or were pain-free or experiencing much less pain. Then instruct yourself to act as if this image were true.

Symbolic imagery

Envision a symbol that represents your chronic pain, such as a loud, irritating noise or a painfully bright light bulb. Gradually reduce the irritating qualities of this symbol. For example dim the light or reduce the volume of the noise, thereby reducing the pain.

Positive Imagery

Focus your attention on a pleasant place that you could imagine going - the beach, mountains, etc. - where you feel carefree, safe and relaxed. Think back to our Happy Place exercise.

Counting

Silent counting is a good way to distract the mind from pain. You might count breaths, count ceiling tiles, or simply conjure up mental images and count them.

Pain Movement

Move chronic back pain from one area of your body to another, where the pain is easier to cope with. For example, mentally move your chronic back pain slowly into your hand, or even out of your hand into the air. Think back to our Moving Tension exercise.

Control Panel

Imagine yourself shrinking down into your body and going into your brain, where there is a control panel. Search the control panel for the dial which changes your sensation of pain. Before turning the dial down, it is always a good idea to up it one notch, if you feel able, for a second or two before turning down to the sensation to an acceptable pain level for yourself.

EXERCISE AND ACTIVITY

Being physically active in general may also help with chronic pain - though, of course the activity must be congruent with your medical condition. Heavy sprints and damaged knees are not a good mix! Speak to your physician or trainer for advice. Rest used to be recommend for almost all chronic conditions. These days, one to three days rest is recognised as being enough, then it is best to return to whatever activities are suitable. Even taking a short walk can be beneficial, both mentally and physically.

Aside from the strengthening the body-mind connection, exercise also means we meet new people, extend our social circle, and become involved in wider activities. They may also give us a forum to share problems or issues and get extra advice and support, all of which are very helpful when dealing with stress or depression.

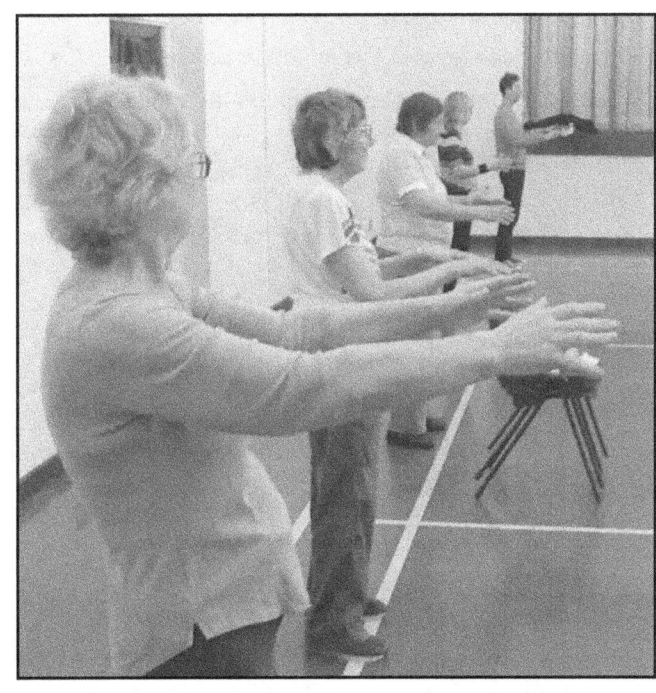

COPING WITH GRIEF

Grief is the intense emotional response we experience following a loss in our lives. That loss may be bereavement, it may be the end of a relationship, it could even be the discovery that we have a serious illness. Grief will manifest in both physical and emotional ways, with reactions ranging from crying, feeling sick, shaking, through to guilt, despair, anger and confusion. It will touch all of us at some point in our lives, none of us are immune to it. It can be overwhelming, it may inhibit us or it may drive us into behaviour that is out of the norm.

It may be helpful to think of grief as an actual, physical wound. Imagine we have a deep, infected cut on our arm, for example. We first have to acknowledge the wound. We next have to begin cleaning out the infection before the wound can begin to heal. We must then allow the wound time to heal, during which it will gradually become less tender and painful. Eventually, the wound will be healed, though it may leave a scar. It's a rather general comparison but at least fixes in our minds the idea that all wounds will eventually heal, given time and given the right approach.

You have probably heard about the Seven Stages of Grief model. These are listed as:

Shock - an initial paralysis at hearing the bad news
Denial - refusal to accept the situation
Anger - an outpouring of bottled-up emotion
Bargaining - looking for a way to change the situation
Depression - realisation of the situation
Testing - seeking realistic solutions
Acceptance - moving forward.

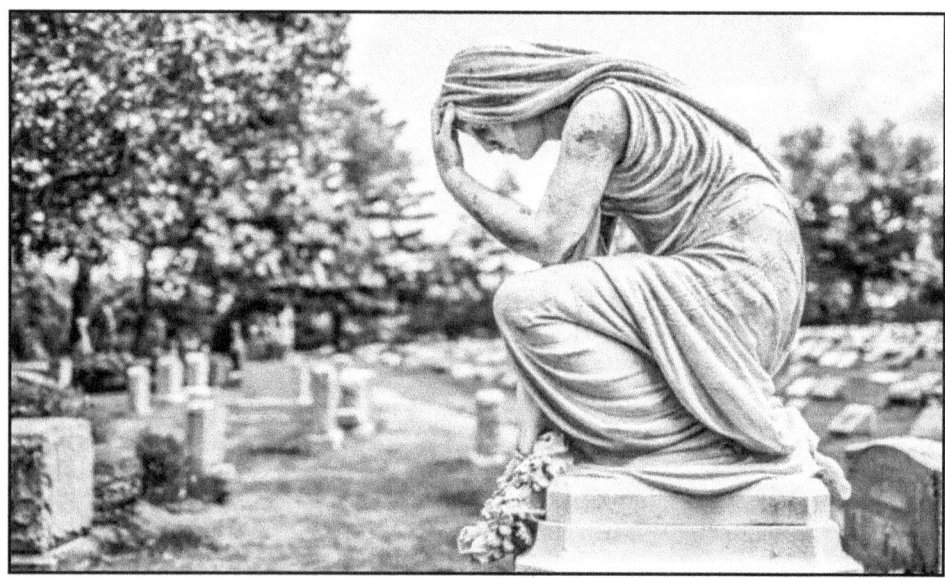

A common problem with the above cycle is that people get stuck in one stage. So a person may become stuck in the denial phase, never moving on from the position of not accepting the situation. That may result in a person pretending to go to work when they have lost their job. Or a bereaved parent might keep a room as it is, "in case the person comes back."

It may be that a particular stage is experienced but not expressed - anger may be bottled up inside, for example. These stages need not be linear, people can move backwards as well as forwards. We may even get stuck in a loop, cycling between anger and depression, which, in itself, becomes a form of avoidance. In that sense, we have to complete one stage before moving onto the next.

There are no one size fits all guidelines to dealing with grief, it is such a personal experience. One thing, however, seems to work across the board and that is emotional release.

EMOTIONAL RELEASE

Many of the Seven Stages involve denying or repressing our grief in some way. In order to process our emotional distress and move through it, we need to learn to express our emotions in a healthy way. The first step is learning to recognize and accept our feelings as they come and go.

Self awareness will be developed through many of the practices in this book - our breath and body work, mindfulness practices and so on. In terms of grief, we could take the Quiet Sitting practice and use it to scan ourselves first for physical tension and then to examine our emotional state. Do you feel angry? Bitter?

Loss brings many emotions with it. You may not have had a good relationship with the deceased, which brings feelings of guilt. You may hold someone responsible in some way, which creates anger. Acknowledge the emotion and feel it in your body, without judgement. Accept that it is okay and perfectly natural to feel this way. Note the physical sensation that the emotion brings - tension, perhaps, or increased heart rate.

Once we have established our inner feelings, we can work to express them. The goal is to

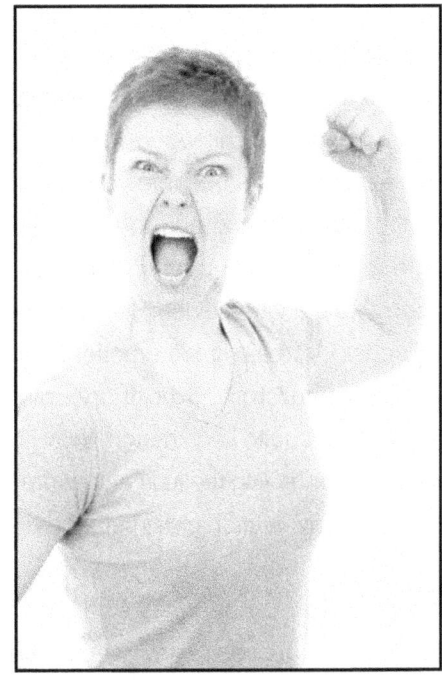

move the energy of the emotion through and out of the body so we can let it go. This expression must be honest. True healing only occurs when body and mind integrate, so express the emotion on the bodily level first.

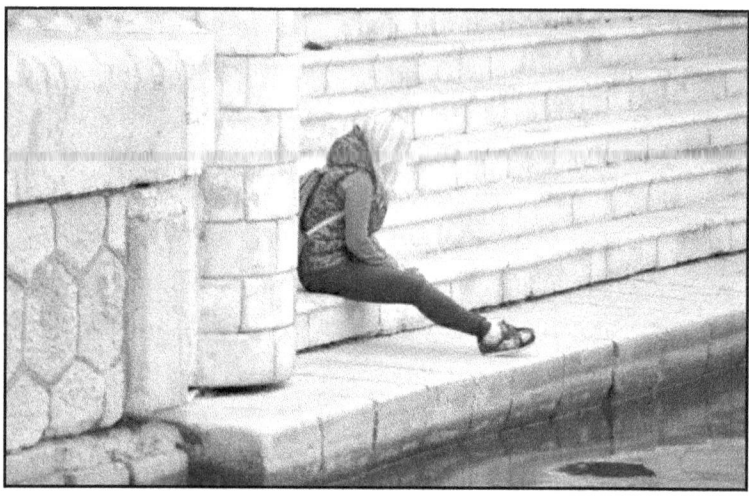

Ask yourself what the emotion you just connected with needs from you? What feels right in this moment? Maybe you feel the need to cry, scream into a pillow, go for run, dance, hit a punching bag, or simply find a quiet place out in nature. Whatever feels cathartic in that moment, do it. Allow yourself to grieve.

As I wrote this book, Monty Python star Terry Jones passed away. The day that the news was announced, there was a TV interview with his long-time friend and colleague Michael Palin. Not unreasonably, he became very emotional during the interview and had to take a minute out. The interesting thing was that Palin then said "sorry" to the interviewer. He felt he had to apologise for expressing his emotions. Maybe this is a very English thing - stiff upper lip and all that? I found it quite sad, though. Why should we apologise for having feelings and expressing them, particularly in such circumstances?

Of course, there may be times when we have to plough on, regardless of how we are feeling. But this constant repression of emotion only leads to problems. Expressing anger, grief, frustration, even love and affection, have typically been frowned upon in some circles, especially for men. A sobering thought in light of the fact that suicide remains the most common cause of death for men aged 20-49 in the UK. So allow yourself to grieve, to express whichever emotion you are feeling. We should never feel ashamed of our feelings, nor should we judge others for expressing theirs.

You may also find it helpful to write your experiences down. Writing gives our internal world a voice. It helps us to process and make sense of what is happening within us and around us. It can also help us gain perspective, allows us a a way of detaching ourselves a little from the situation.

The final step in the grief cycle is to reset ourselves back to our usual state of being and wellness. Make some time available to spend on yourself. Do something you find relaxing, anything that will help bring you back into enjoying life's simple pleasures. Also allow yourself item to grieve. Nothing here needs to be rushed and it is important to re-emphasise that nothing here is about suppressing grief, or feeling that your are somehow being "bad" for feeling the emotions that you do.

Be prepared for occasional lapses too, if that is the correct word. You may have to deal with a deceased person's personal effects. You may find yourself taking the dog lead from its hook in preparation for taking the deceased dog for a walk. Incidentally, I'm not one to downplay the feeling of loss we can experience through the death of a pet. Of course, our pets are "just animals" but they do become a big part of our lives.

Many things may trigger a return of grief. About a year after my mother's death, I was in a music store. A song came over the loudspeaker that had been played at her funeral, and I was totally and unexpectedly overwhelmed. Again, learn to accept the emotion and do what is necessary to release it.

Also, take the time to remember the good things about the deceased. Looking through old photos or the like can be a comforting experience, we remember the good times we had. Talking with others, sharing our memories and feelings or speaking to a counsellor will also help us process our grief. In the end, however deep the pain, we have to learn to let go.

LETTING GO

There are some other methods we can use to help us move through our grief. If the death was unexpected, we may have things unsaid, or feel that we did not have time to say *goodbye*. Closure is a powerful part of the healing process. One simple exercise is to write a letter to the deceased. Tell them all the things you'd like them to hear, or perhaps never had the chance to say previously. Hand write the letter and be totally honest in what you write. Once you have finished, find a space outside where you can set a match to the letter and let it burn. Allow the embers to float away, visualise them carrying your words to the deceased.

Learning to let go can also help us in other situations. As well a grief, we experience anger in our lifetime, perhaps the result of some type of bad behaviour towards us (something exacerbated by social media, in my view!). It may be that we refuse to accept the ending of a relationship, we are unable to move forward with our lives. Learning to let go of someone we've built a deep connection with is understandably difficult. However, in many cases, it's necessary to let go in order to unlock our future life.

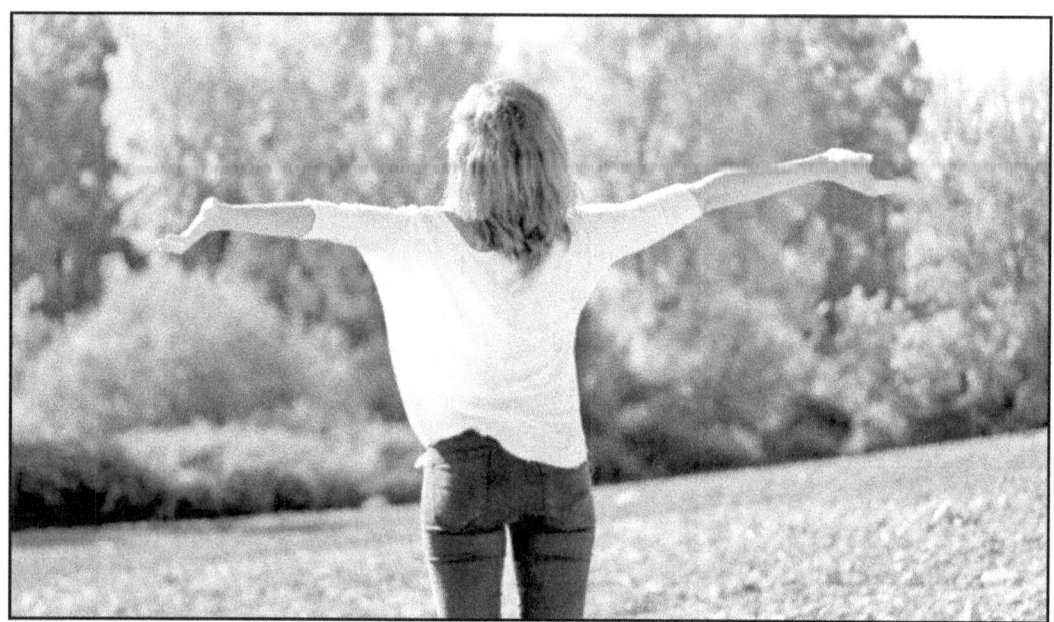

We all like to hold on to things, situations and circumstances because there's comfort in familiarity, even when it's rooted in a negative experience. Sometimes, we use the past to justify our current decision-making, another reason why we don't want to let go. Changing this outlook involves controlling the meaning we attach to events in our lives. This process again involves recognising the emotions we are feeling, as in the previous exercise and, if necessary, releasing them.

If the situation is a relationship break-up, it may also be helpful to think of both sides of the story. Try to see the situation from the other person's point of view, understand why they came to the decision that they did. From there, you might also try to look at this person from the same place of compassion that you did when you were happy together. Let go of the expectations of what you think needs to happen right now to ease your pain and focus on gratitude for what you once shared. This should help you reduce the anger you feel toward the other person and allow you to appreciate what you gained from the relationship.

After that, work on forgiveness for getting so caught up in the drama of your personal life and allowing your anger and resentment to hurt you and hold you back. Realise that this is an opportunity chance to grow and move on to the next phase of your life.

Learning how to let go is not as hard as it may seem. Unwanted things will happen, but we cannot change the past and refusing to let go will not bring someone you care about back. Continuing to hold on only hurts our emotional and physical state. Face what has happened, accept that you can't change it and move on.

This isn't only about accepting situations, though. We also have to accept people for who they are rather than who we may wish them to be. This means we sometimes have to forgive people who aren't even sorry, to accept an apology you'll never receive. That takes some strength and seems very unfair, but holding onto resentment while the other person happily moves on with their life, only hurts you.

Learn to forgive yourself, too! We don't always make the right decisions, we upset people, we do things wrong. What's done is done, the important thing is we learn from those mistakes and try not to repeat them in the future. Dwelling on "what ifs" and "if onlys" is a waste of time and imagination - both can be put to better use!

EMOTIONAL RELEASE EXERCISE

We should also not neglect the physical aspects of emotional tension. Earlier we discussed how emotional issues can manifest as muscular tensions, from shallow to deep. You might find it beneficial to run through a complete Selective Tension exercise to assist in letting go, too. Here's how it works.

Set aside a time and place, a warm, comfortable environment. Run through the previous

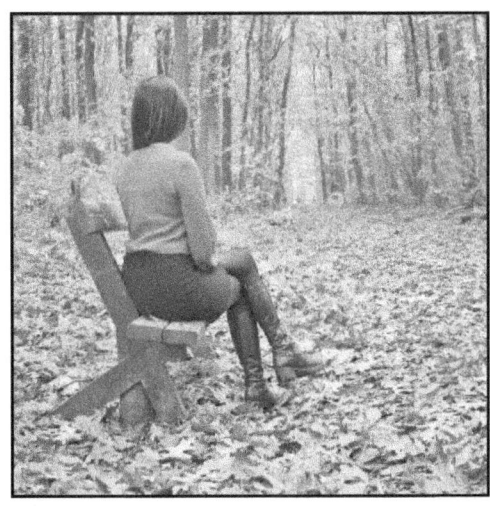

Selective Tension routine as normal to start, working with any surface muscular tension.

Next, we work a little deeper. Bring your grief to mind ands see how it effects you physically. Feel which parts of your body react to the grief. Are your shoulders hunched? Do you feel tension in the stomach area? Inhale, increase the tension in that place and hold for at least 30 seconds. Exhale and release. Let the emotion go with the tension. If you cry, or shout, that's fine, it's all a release. When done, have a hot drink, wrap a blanket round your shoulders and sit quietly for a while

Letting go of more complex or intense experiences will likely involve deeper work, such as therapy or similar. Dealing with issues of PTSD or deep seated emotional trauma are best carried out under professional guidance. The goods news is that, now matter how bad things seem, they will get better if we accept help.

CHAPTER EIGHT
MANAGING CONFLICT AND FEAR

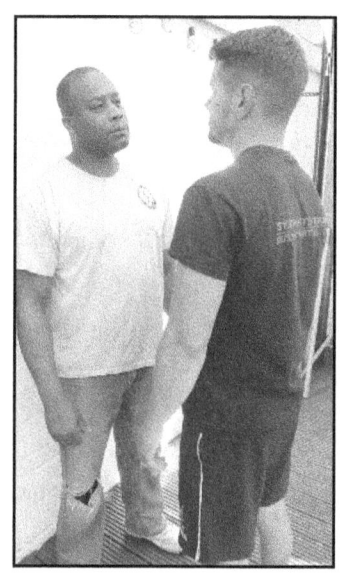

Fear and aggression are universal human emotions and can be a major cause of stress. That may be an immediate stress, if we are confronted with an angry person. It might be an anticipatory fear, such as the anxiety caused by having to make a speech. The fear may even relate to events that occurred many years ago, in the case of trauma and phobias.

Conflict is wide in scope and difficult to avoid. It may be a couple's tiff, It might be an argument over a parking space, it could be an aggressive or pushy work colleague. At a more dangerous level, it could be a potentially violent confrontation. Even going on social media these days seems to lead to conflict, judging by the needles arguments that rage over even the most trivial of matters. The sheer bile and bitterness on display on-line has to make you wonder if people have always been this angry or does the anonymity of the situation encourage such bad behaviour?

On-line bullying has become a real issue for young people. It's easy for an adult to say *ignore it, switch off* but not always so easy for young people to deal with the situation. Fortunately, schools and others are much more active these days when it comes to anti-bullying measures, whether in the virtual or the real world.

Tackling issues of bullying, intimidation and violence is another large topic, with a range of options available, from assertiveness training to self defence classes. From our stress angle, let's first look at how we can recognise when a problem is arising.

CONFLICT RESOLUTION

The better we can recognise stress in ourselves, the easier we can spot it in others. If your work involves members of the public, whether in a services or retail environment, you may occasionally have to deal with difficult situations. Spotting when people are becoming stressed will help you to manage the situation and steer it to a successful outcome. The same applies to any potentially stressful encounter, even something like a business negotiation.

People are often surprised to hear that over 90% of personal communication is non-verbal. Half of that is through body language and the remainder is in tone of voice. Only a small percentage of communication relates to the actual words used. It is virtually impossible for humans to not display something of their internal or psychological state in their physical being.

Body language is the study and understanding of what these physical signs indicate. Many of these reactions occur without conscious thought, so they give a true insight as to a person's intent. Being able to read body language gives us a very useful tool when dealing with people. It is a huge topic in itself,

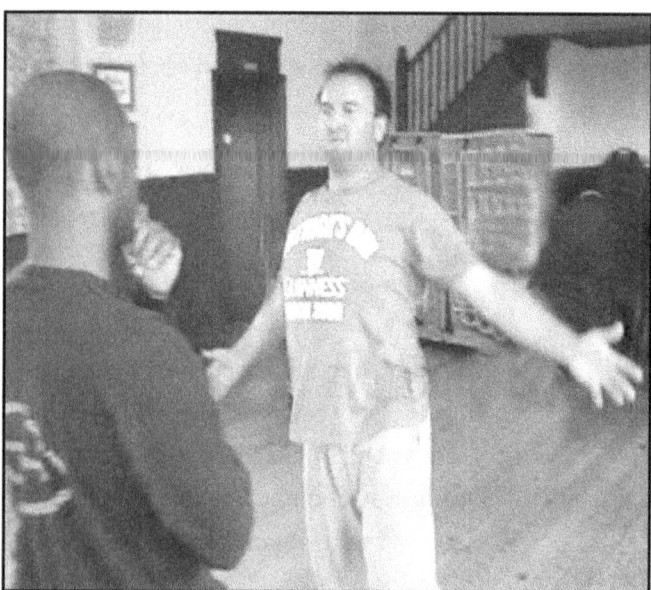

STRESS INDICATORS

The first signs we will look for are known as pacifiers. These are actions taken by people as they begin to feel stressed, in order to calm themselves down. One of the main actions is touching and stroking, particularly the neck or face. Some speculate that touching the neck, particularly just under the chin is an unconscious response to increased blood pressure. A similar move may be to adjust the tie knot or to tug on the collar. Men tend to do this more than women, who tend to cover the neck rather than stroke it.

with many layers. For our purposes, the biggest single indicator when observing behaviour is to determine whether a person is stressed or at ease. We may think of stress as anger, fear, lust, anxiety. A person at ease, is happy, confident, relaxed. In general we can broadly divide every emotional state into comfort or discomfort and both will exhibit their own particular physical manifestations. We can do this by watching out for stress indicators.

A person interrogating a suspect, for example, will be watching for stress indicators that might be a sign of lying. A sales person will seek to establish rapport with a customer, to make them feel at ease and hopefully more receptive to the sales pitch. Indicators range from the quite obvious to the more subtle. This is an overview of behaviours to watch for.

As far as the face goes, people may rub their forehead, massage an earlobe or lick the lips. Arms and legs are another area to watch. Crossed arms can be an indicator of the "self hug", particularly if the hands rub the arms. The "leg cleanse" is a common movement, too. People place palms on their upper thigh and rub down towards the knee.

Let's now take a run through the main body areas and discuss the signals that each may give away. Again, this is quite a brief overview of this topic, but is enough to give you some good tips and a starting point for further study.

BREATHING

Breathing and sound are another good indicator

of pacifying behaviour. People may puff out their cheeks, then exhale loudly. Whistling is another calming activity. Stress can even cause excessive yawning, a response to the mouth becoming dry. Of course, shortness and shallowness of breath will often indicate nervousness, so listen to how a person breathes, or works to adjust their breathing.

FEET & LEGS

The feet, surprisingly perhaps, are known as the most honest part of the body! The zoologist Desmond Morris observed that the feet reveal our feelings more honestly than any other part of the body. People in a good mood may jiggle or bounce their feet. Lifting the toes or rocking up and down is also the sign of a good mood. We are so happy that gravity can't affect us! Jittery feet, or foot tapping, may indicate impatience.

Foot direction is important, too. When you see a pair talking, observe which direction the feet point in. We tend to turn towards something we like and away from something we don't. If one foot keeps turning away, then back again, it may be a sign that person wants to exit the conversation. This applies even when seated. It can also be accompanied by a forward lean and a knee clasp.

Legs are also a great indicator of mood, they are often used in territorial displays. Feet and legs tend to splay out in confrontational situations, perhaps in an attempt to increase "size" or space occupied. Standing with feet together tends to give a more passive signal. Crossing legs when standing is often a sign of comfort (or needing the loo!). It compromises

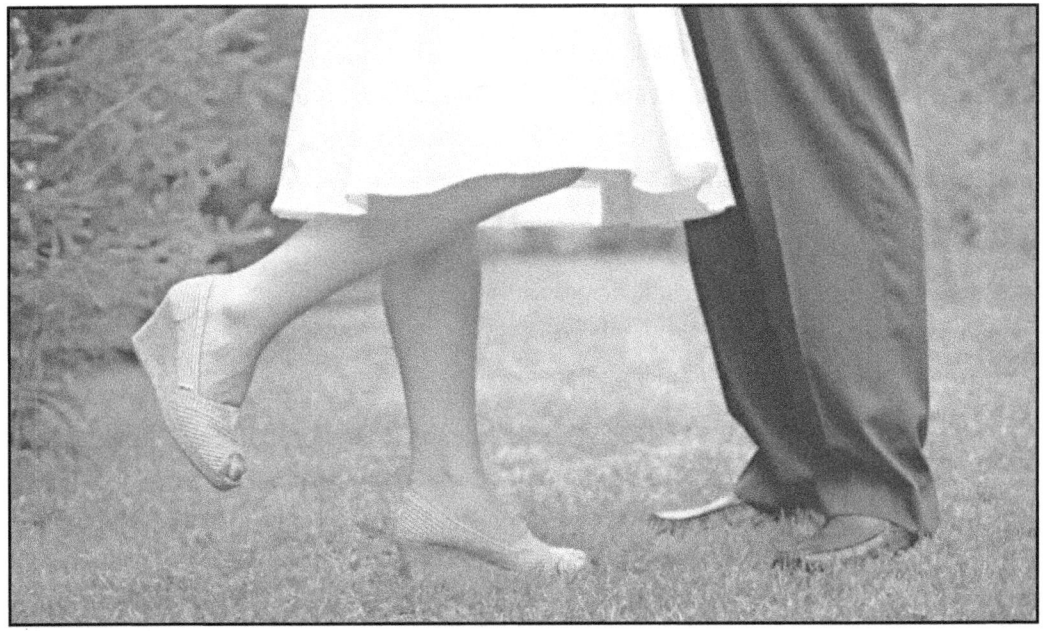

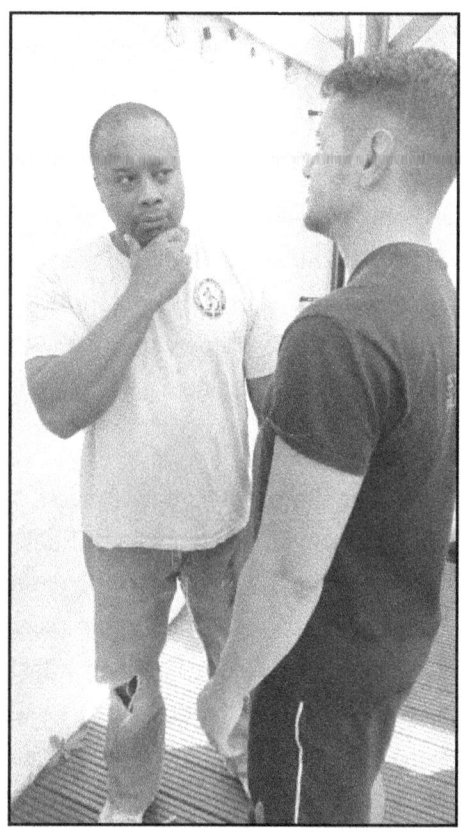

our vital organs – heart, lungs, kidneys, etc. Perhaps for this reason the usual behaviour of a stressed torso is to create distance. Have you ever seen someone in a social situation being "chatted up" by a person they don't like? This is a prime place to observe the "torso lean." The person feels they cannot get up and walk away but the body will lean away from the offending party.

Another version of this is blading. This is where the torso is turned at a slight angle from the perceived threat. Fronting is a more aggressive action. The chest is puffed out, the arms splayed, a classic territorial display. It may even lead to chest bumping and what has become known as the *monkey dance*, where two people want to show they are willing to fight but might not really actually want to yet!

our balance, so is not a stance usually seen in a stressful situation. Done in a pair, it shows that the people are at ease with each other. If a stranger enters the situation, the legs will probably uncross.

The seated cross leg position is a little different. Direction becomes important again. A thigh can be used as a barrier. However if the knee faces the other way, this shows a person at ease with the other party.

TORSO

If you think about out, the torso contains most of

ARMS

The shoulder is the most mobile joint in the body. Correspondingly, our arms tend to be very expressive. We use our arms as barriers, we use them to welcome, we use them to occupy space. Covering the torso with the arms may be pacifying behaviour, it can also be a method of shielding or blocking. Chest shielding is generally more prominent in women, for obvious reasons, perhaps, but men will exhibit the same. Crossing an arm over the body to fiddle with a cufflink, for example.

.Sometimes the shoulders rise slowly. This is

known as *turtling* almost as though the person is trying to withdraw into their shell. It's usually a sign of discomfort or of not wanting to be associated with whatever is going on.

Shielding by crossing the arms is usually an indicator of dislike or discomfort. Buttoning up a jacket may show a similar thing. We have already mentioned the other version of crossing arms, the self hug, as a pacifying gesture. By contrast, when happy or joyful we tend to raise our arms, as though defying gravity. As a rough guide, think hands up happy, hands down, sad.

FACE

The most expressive part of our body and the one we observe the most in order to gauge another person's thought or emotions. The number of human facial expressions is estimated as over ten thousand. For the most part, they are universal across all cultures. Sad people look the same sad all around the world!

We can, to a degree, control our facial muscles, so the face may not always be the best indicator. Having said that, there is something called micro-expressions that we can watch out for. Micro-expressions are very brief, involuntary expressions that appear on a person's face according to the emotions being experienced. They usually occur as fast as 1/15 to 1/25 of a second. Unlike regular expressions, they are difficult to fake. There are seven universal micro-expressions:

disgust, anger, fear, sadness, happiness, surprise and contempt.

I'm sure you are able to recognise each of those - the brows knit for anger, the lips turn up for a smile for happiness, down for sadness and so on. The trick is to catch these expressions as they occur. A person attempting to mask their emotions will quickly regain control of the facial muscles to present whatever it is they wish to project. However, that little flash of honesty may give the game away, so watch out for them!

If we go back to our idea of comfort and stress, it is generally true that negative emotions bring tension with them. Brows furrow, jaws clench, nostrils flare, lips press together. When we are happy, our faces tend to "open" more. We smile, our eyes widen, the eyebrows raise and so on. These are all very obvious indicators of state of mind.

MIRRORING AND RAPPORT

Having spotted the beginnings of stress in a person, how do we put them at ease? We have to work to establish what is known as rapport, to help the person see that we are on their side and not in opposition to them. One way to achieve this is through mirroring. The basic idea is that two people in synch usually mirror each other's body language. This is the opposite of the shielding or foot direction work we discussed earlier. People who are in synch typically face each other, draw close, leave their

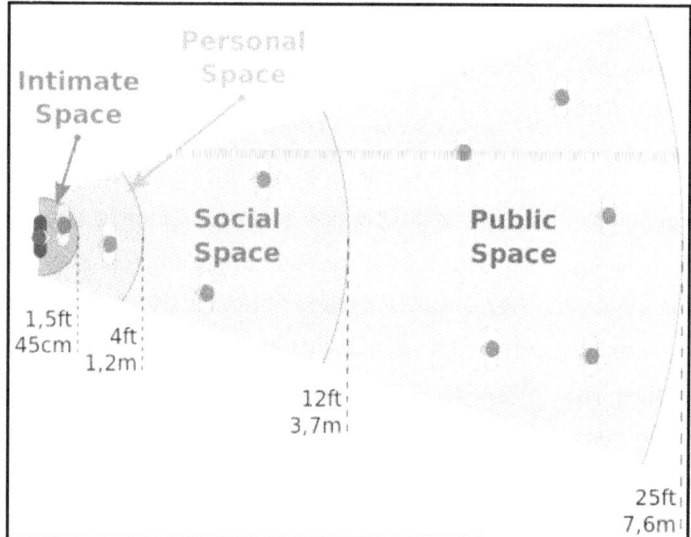

Proxemics, a term was coined in 1963 by cultural anthropologist Edward T. Hall. There are four zones within his model.

- public space is categorised as being at least 12 feet away.
- social space is within the range of 4-12 feet.
- personal space is defined as a range of 1.5-4 feet.
- intimate space is from touch to 1.5 feet.

The distinctions are fairly obvious. Around friends and family, we feel no discomfort at being at intimate distance. In another situation, a stranger moving even to within personal space, may trigger stress. There are other factors to take into account, cultural and environmental mostly, but the general rule remains - crowd someone and they will feel stressed.

Another consideration is how you approach a person. Imagine marching directly up to someone while maintaining unwavering eye contact with them. Chances are that may be seen as confrontational! Instead, approach slightly from the side. From there, work to establish a common point of view - as you reach the person, adjust position so that your direction of vision is the same as theirs. In other words, you are both looking at the same thing. This establishes a much stronger feeling in the

torso uncovered and so on. You can try this out with a friend Talk to them and as you chat, slowly adopt the same posture as the other person. Add in an open expression, a smile, tilt your head slightly. Maintain eye contact, nod, raise your eyebrows. These are all signs that you agree with and are comfortable with this person.

Once you've tried that, repeat but this time do the reverse. Close off, cross your arms, look away frequently, angle your body. Ask your partner how each feels to them. Always be aware that mirroring should be a subtle process. Too overt and it just looks weird, so causing stress!

When it comes to establishing rapport, something else to be aware of is personal space. We have quite distinct zones of comfort around us. The study of these spaces is called person that you are working with them.

Understanding motivation is another key component of managing confrontation. Why is a person acting the way they are? Perhaps they have a genuine grievance. It could be they are under the influence of alcohol or drugs. Peer pressure is something else to consider - a person may react quite differently alone than when with a group of friends or in front of their partner.

Think about how you establish a connection. When you first approach, also ask the person their name, for example. Talking calmly, especially asking questions, allows us to move closer. Now we can begin to build empathy - understand the other person's point of view. If possible, get them to understand yours, or even to extend you some sympathy. *If I don't ask you to do this my boss may fire me!*

Always be sure to explain yourself - make the details of the situation clear and your own role within it. If appropriate, explain the advantage to the person for doing what you ask them to do. *If you stay here, you may get bumped into, there's a crowd of people coming through. I wouldn't want you to spill your drink.*

Be firm but fair, be open and confident, do not show fear or aggression. Be clear in your aims but not totally inflexible. Also bear in mind what we said earlier about tone of voice. How you say is as important as what you say. Also, should the situation escalate, be prepared to take action, whether that be to create space, to withdraw from the situation, to call for help or to take direct action (if trained and appropriate).

As we mentioned, there are any number of potential conflict situations we may face on a daily basis. It is impossible to give hard and fast rules to cover every scenario, but the above guidelines will at least give you good start point. Above all, remain as calm as possible. However provoked or justified you feel, avoid becoming drawn into to the argument.

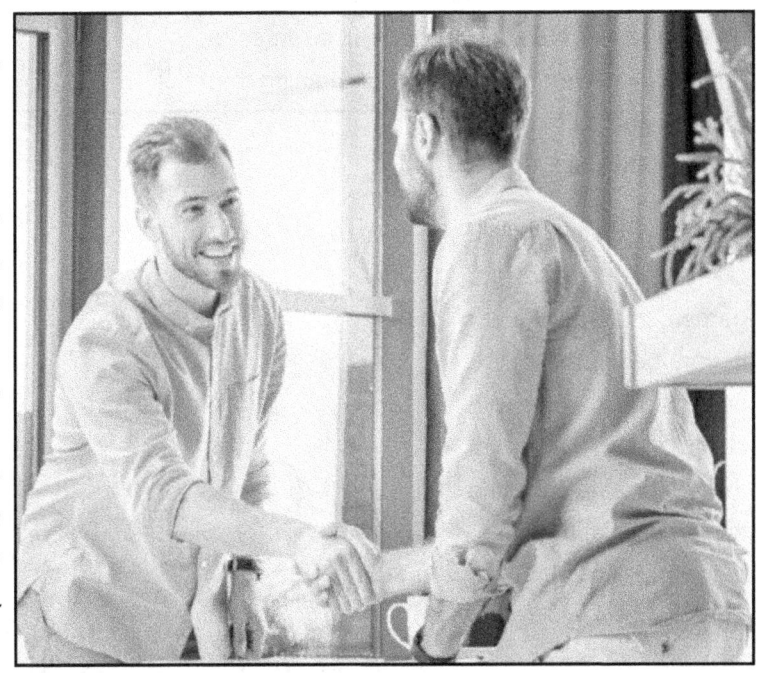

FEAR CONTROL

Fear is a perfectly normal emotion and, as we mentioned before, can be very useful. However there is also a saying about something making *a good servant but a bad master*. In that respect, if we allow fear to control every aspect of our lives we are likely not only cutting ourselves off from potentially positive experiences but also putting our mental health at risk.

Some fears come and go in an instant - we catch sight of a garden hose and think it's a snake! We jump, laugh at our silliness and move on. Other fears stay longer. In the case of fears resulting from trauma, they may be with us for years or even decades. Phobias are deep-seated fears, perhaps extending back to something that happened in our childhood. In both cases, we need to tackle the root of the fear in order to release ourselves from its grip - something that may take some time and professional help.

Fear can be instinctive (as in the case of the garden snake above) or it can be learned. We have to be careful with children, in that we want them to be safe but at the same time instilling too much fear at a young age may lead to problems later on.

When it comes to more everyday fears, many of the methods already described will help - breathing to unlock our freeze reaction, exercises to release muscular tension and so on. However there are some additional exercises and methods we can practice in order to help manage our fears.

Just one other note - fear can manifest itself in many different ways. If I ask you to imagine a scared person, you will perhaps think of someone holding their hands over their face, screaming and shaking. However fear can prompt people into aggressive behaviour, even violence, as well as leading them into lying, stealing, or into those types of compensation actions we spoke of before. Learning to see fear as the root of stressed or abnormal behaviour can help us either deal with our own, or another persons issues.

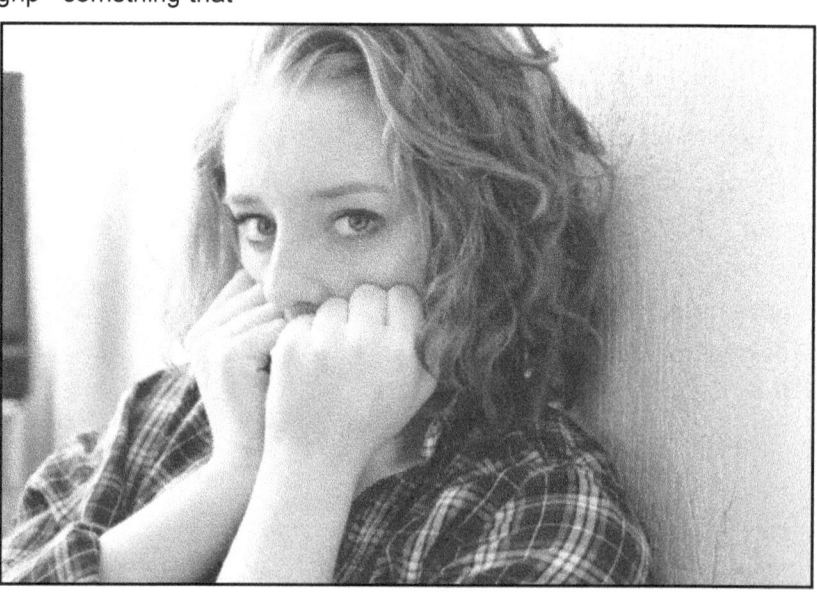

Immediate physical dangers aside, fear is an illusion. It is a construct of our minds, a response to some imagined situation. We might call this type of fear *anticipatory* and it tends to be pervasive and damaging. Because of this fear, we don't apply for that job. We don't write that book because we're worried what people will think. We avoid relationships because we're scared of getting hurt. Our fear becomes a security blanket, we can stay safe in its warm grasp. Throwing the blanket away exposes us to the scary world! But throw it away we must if we are to lead a stress free and happy life.

HORMESIS

The best method I've personally found for overcoming anticipatory fears to give ourselves a small dose of fear, and learn how to manage it. We can then increase the dose slightly, so progressing until we are able to cope with the full-blown fear. The scientific term for this is *hormesis* - using the correct level of stress in order to allow an organism to develop. This is in contrast to the "in at the deep end" approach. Some of you may have had a similar experience to mine; as a kid I was not very confident in water. The PE teacher's answer to this was to have the scared kids literally thrown in at the deep end of the pool, to splutter and sink! It didn't work for me, or any of the others. Perhaps it works for some but we are going to take a different approach.

When undergoing inoculation, it is crucial that we have a coping mechanism to help us deal with that dose of fear. This method is not a case of "toughing it out," all that generally achieves is learning how to mask the fear, to hide it away. While their may be a time and place for the "stiff upper lip," this is not it. We must confront our fear on some level and learn truly overcome it, not just pretend it isn't there.

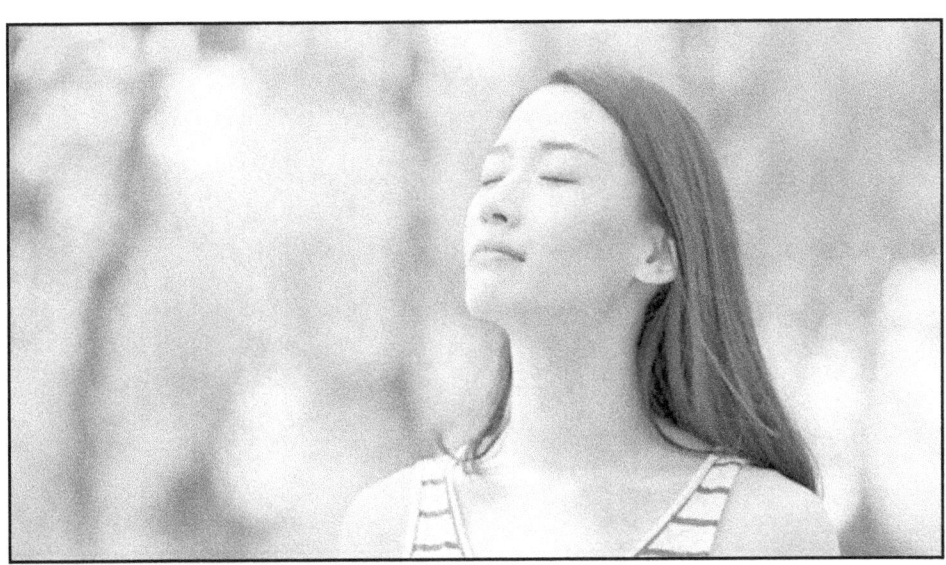

BREATH HOLDS AND RECOVERY

The main coping mechanism we use to overcome our stress response in this method is breathing . Specifically, we are gong to use the Burst Breathing method mentioned earlier.

Burst, or recovery breathing, is where we inhale nose and quickly exhale mouth. The breath is shallow and short, a panting-type breath. A good way to learn this technique is through breath holds. In effect, we hold the breath for as long as we can, release, then go into Burst Breathing to recover. Before we do, just a reminder that if you have blood pressure issues, check first with your doctor before practicing breath holds. Holding the breath can lead to a rise in blood pressure if there is a lot of tension in the body, so it is best to have a good ground in the Circular Breathing method before trying this.

When holding the breath, keep the body as relaxed as possible. Do not take a big inhale by expanding the chest and lifting the shoulders. Simply take a normal, relaxed inhale to about 80% of your capacity. Of course, only carry out the practice in a safe environment. If you do begin to feel a bit lightheaded or stressed, immediately release the breath and go into Burst Breathing.

Sit in a comfortable position and begin with Circular Breaths. After a short time, take an inhale and hold it. Remember, chest and

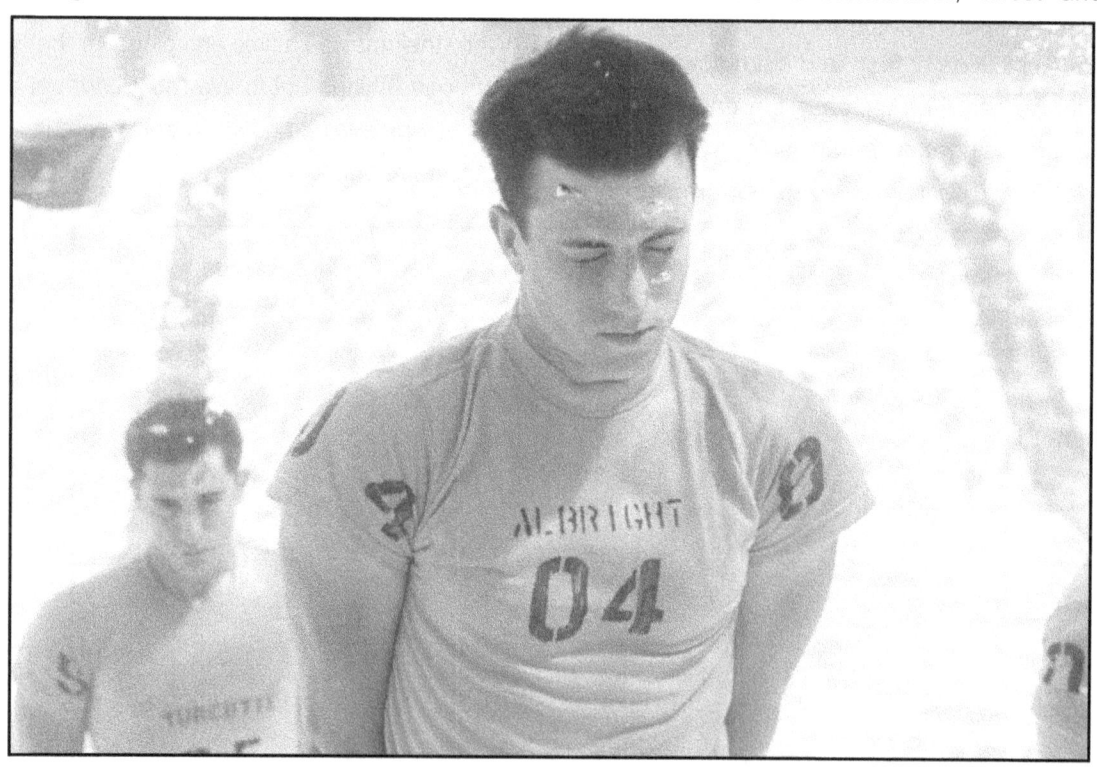

shoulders relaxed. After a time, you will naturally want to release the breath and start breathing again. Resist this temptation. Feel the sensation in the body - is there an area which is tense? Work to relax it, either by movement or with selective tension.

After another time the sensation will return, maybe a little stronger. If you can, resist it again. Relax yourself physically and psychologically. Finally, when you can hold no longer, release the breath. Immediately go into Burst Breathing, short, sharp inhale - exhales. Then slowly lengthen the breathes until they are back to normal length and any stress or tension is gone.

When you come out of a breath hold, you may want to try and fill your lungs with as much air as possible. Avoid the temptation, keep the breathing shallow, this will bring you back to stability much quicker. It's a little like the advice given to people who have water after wandering in the desert for a few days - don't gulp, take little sips!

Once you have the idea, you can work the same process but hold on an exhale (with the lungs 80% empty). This is a little more challenging but very beneficial.

The Breath Holds themselves are are form of hormesis. We are introducing a level of stress into the body in order to learn how to cope with it. The stress level is entirely under our control - we choose when to begin breathing again.

Breath Holds are a good indicator of general health. Some practitioners even use them as a diagnostic too. They are also an excellent method of learning to deal with fear. This is because not being able to breathe is a primal human fear - it triggers our fear of death very quickly. If we can control fear at such a primal level, we have a much greater chance of overcoming "lesser" fears.

There are entire methods of development built around breath holds - most of them stemming from the Russian health systems. Others use them in endurance feats, the most notable being in the sport of free diving. This involves submerging yourself in depths of water, with no oxygen, and seeing who can stay down the longest! The worlds record for an unassisted free dive is 11 minutes, 35 seconds for men and 8 minutes, 23 seconds for women, which shows what remarkable feats humans are capable of when our minds and body work perfectly in tune.

Our needs are somewhat more modest! Having said that, if your practice breath holds regularly, you will gradually extend your hold time. This, aside from stress reduction benefits, will also develop your willpower, strengthen the lungs and increase your recovery time. Now let's look at how we can use BB as a coping mechanism in our fear inoculation process.

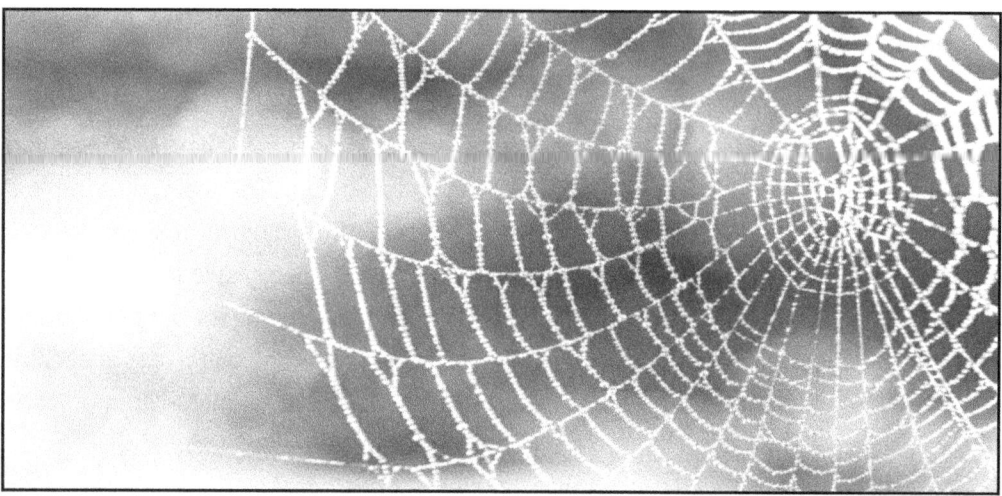

FEAR INOCULATION STAGES

Let's take a very common fear - spiders. Does even reading that word give you a physical feeling? Did you shiver a little, perhaps? Good, we have already started!

Each stage in the FI process has three components - the trigger, the reaction and the coping mechanism. The latter is usually the same in each case, and is in proportion to the strength of reaction. So a mild reaction, such as feeling a bit uneasy, might call for a little bit of Burst Breathing. A stronger reaction, such as a panic attack, may call for an additional Quiet Sitting session and/ or some type of exercise or movement. Do whatever you need to do in order to bring your body systems back to normal.

The trigger is simply a graded level of exposure to the cause of the fear or phobia. It is progressive, you can think of it as a ladder, and it is okay to go back down a step or two if we need too. Let's look at how an arachnaphobia trigger sequence might work, along with how to monitor reaction and use a control mechanism.

Trigger One
What image does the word *spider* conjure in your mind?

Reaction - note your physical response to the image. Understand that your body is reacting to something that is totally made up in your mind. Note if there is any tension in your body - are your shoulders hunched, perhaps?

How is your breathing? Has it sped up a little? Control mechanism - wiggle your shoulders around a little to get rid of the tension. Work some Burst Breathing to calm it down again.

Trigger Two
Look at a picture of a spider, just a quick glance. Again, and in all the following stages, note reactions and apply your coping mechanism.

Trigger Three
Closely examine the picture of the spider. What is there about it that looks unpleasant? Is there anything that looks nice? The web, perhaps, or colourful markings.

Trigger Four
Watch some footage of a spider, on You-tube or similar. Keep it brief at first. Start with footage of a garden spider building a web.

Trigger Five
Watch several clips of spiders.

Trigger Six
Look at a real spider. You don't have to get too close, and it can be in a controlled environment, such as a zoo or pet shop. Be confident that you have an "escape route" in case you get overwhelmed. Again, examine what it is about the spider that worries you, what is it that might attract you.

Trigger Seven
Get up close to a real spider. Perhaps in the garden, or in a shed.

Trigger Eight
Remove a spider from your house. Use a cup and card, or perhaps one of those new-fangled "bug remover" devices! Monitor your reactions throughout.

Trigger Nine
Handle a spider. Visit a pet shop or similar and see if you can hold a spider in your hand.

This sequence is a rough blueprint to overcoming most types of anticipatory fear. Your fear might be public speaking and perhaps you have to give a wedding speech in a few months time. Apply the same procedure. Begin by imagining yourself giving a speech, then read a speech out loud while alone. Progress to giving the speech to family and friends, work up to speaking in public.

Whatever the issue, there are a few things to bear in mind when working through trigger stages:

You are in control - at each trigger event, you are in full control of the situation. You can call a halt at any time, you can walk away at any time.

Be specific - set very clear goals about what you want to achieve and structure your trigger stages accordingly.

Be realistic - if you are terrified of heights, don't plan to make a parachute jump in a month's time, unless you are very confident!

Don't be too timid - by the same token, do set yourself goals and targets. You may even find you progress more quickly than you thought possible.

Be creative - the above are only guidelines. Find your own methods of setting trigger stages and explore other coping mechanisms (as long as they are positive ones).

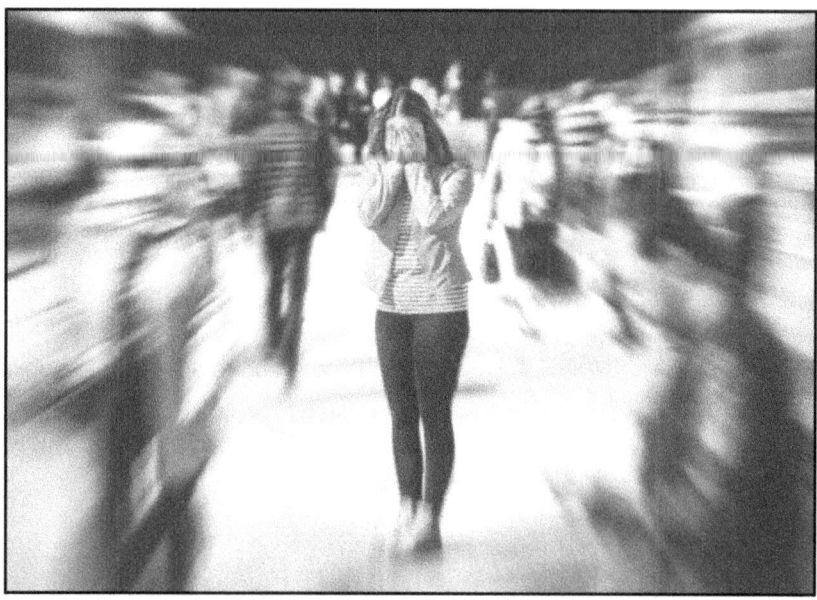

Anticipate setbacks - there are bound to be times when the process becomes difficult. We may even slip back a stage now and then. This is perfectly normal, life is never a nice, even progression. Don't be discouraged, keep on keeping on!

Be kind to yourself - one friend promised himself a treat upon successfully dealing with each trigger stage. Don't be afraid to reward yourself, it might a be a nice meal or a new pair of shoes! Also, be positive about your achievements, don't give in to negativity.

Don't procrastinate - you can do this now! Avoid saying "I'll start that next month," or, "I'm too busy now." Make the time, make the effort. The sooner you start, the sooner you can overcome this fear!

Analyse and monitor - always apply an analytical mindset to the process. Do other factors affect your fear? Is your fear of being a lift increased if the lift is crowded? Is your fear of flying eased by having a friend fly with you?

Understanding - do some research on your fear trigger. Are you scared that your plane will crash? Do you know how a plane works? What are the safety procedures on a flight? Do you know the current safety records for flying?

Develop skills - another saying is *skill is the enemy of fear*. If we have skills in a certain area, we are less likely to be afraid of being in that situation. If water scares you, take some swimming lessons. You can even build this into your trigger stages. If you have trouble dealing with aggressive people, think about taking some self defence training (look for a class that covers the "soft skills" of awareness and conflict management as well as the more physical methods). This, in itself, may also introduce you to a new and fulfilling hobby.

Get support - never be concerned about asking for help from family and friends. You might even seek out support groups or a professional therapist. This might particularly be applicable in cases of deeper set phobias, traumas and PTSD type conditions.

This Fear Inoculation method, combined with some of the other exercises we have covered, will go a long way to reducing those "everyday" fears. The effect is accumulative, too. I've found that confidence in one area increases confidence in others. In effect, we turn our mindset around from negative to positive. Doing so can have a profound effect on how we view the world and, in turn, how the world views us.

CHAPTER NINE
GOING DEEPER

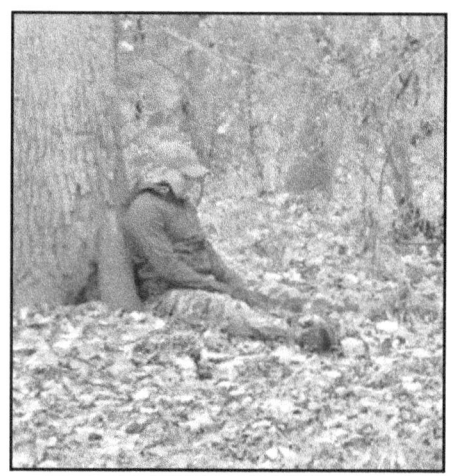

So far we have detailed a range of exercises and strategies that will give you a powerful set of tools for managing the kind of stress that we are up against most days. Hopefully, through instituting some of the strategies discussed, you will also be able to head off a certain amount of stress before it even beings to take hold. However, life is full of unexpected twists and turns and life and we may find ourselves in situations that are beyond our ability to cope. In those cases, we should never be reticent about asking for help, be it professional or from friends and family.

Likewise, we may wish to look more deeply into some of the methods mentioned in this book. Many of the exercises here are described at a basic level, in order to make them accessible and suitable for quick use - there's no need to spend ten years practice to get benefits! Having said that, should you wish to take up any of these disciplines, you will find them a rich source of not only stress management but also wider overall health, fitness and well-being benefits.

I would only caveat that statement by adding that you need to find a good teacher, instructor, practitioner in whatever it is that you are interested in pursuing. There are charlatans in all walks of life, particularly when it comes to some of the more alternative / fringe or less well known activities. Check experience and qualifications where possible, ask around (social media is great for this) and try a few things out before settling on one class or practitioner. Never be afraid to ask questions and don't be taken in by flashy websites or presentation. Let your gut feeling be your guide.

This chapter, then, is a guide to some of the options available should you wish to take things further. It is by no means comprehensive but I hope will give you a good primer as to what is out there. We will also cover a couple of our earlier exercises in greater depth, but let's first start with something mentioned in an earlier chapter, a deeper look at fundamental human needs

MASLOW'S HIERARCHY OF NEEDS

In 1943, the US psychologist Abraham Maslow published a paper called *A Theory of Human Motivation*. In it, he explained that people have five sets of needs, set in a particular order. As each level of need is satisfied, the desire to fulfil the next level is activated. Our primary needs are basic and primitive. Once they are satisfied the needs become more geared to social and ego matters. Perhaps because of this structure the Hierarchy is often represented in pyramid form, see the diagram overleaf.

Maslow classified the bottom four levels of the pyramid as *deficiency needs.* In other words a person does not feel anything if they are met, but becomes anxious if they are not. So needs such as eating, drinking, and sleeping are deficiency needs.

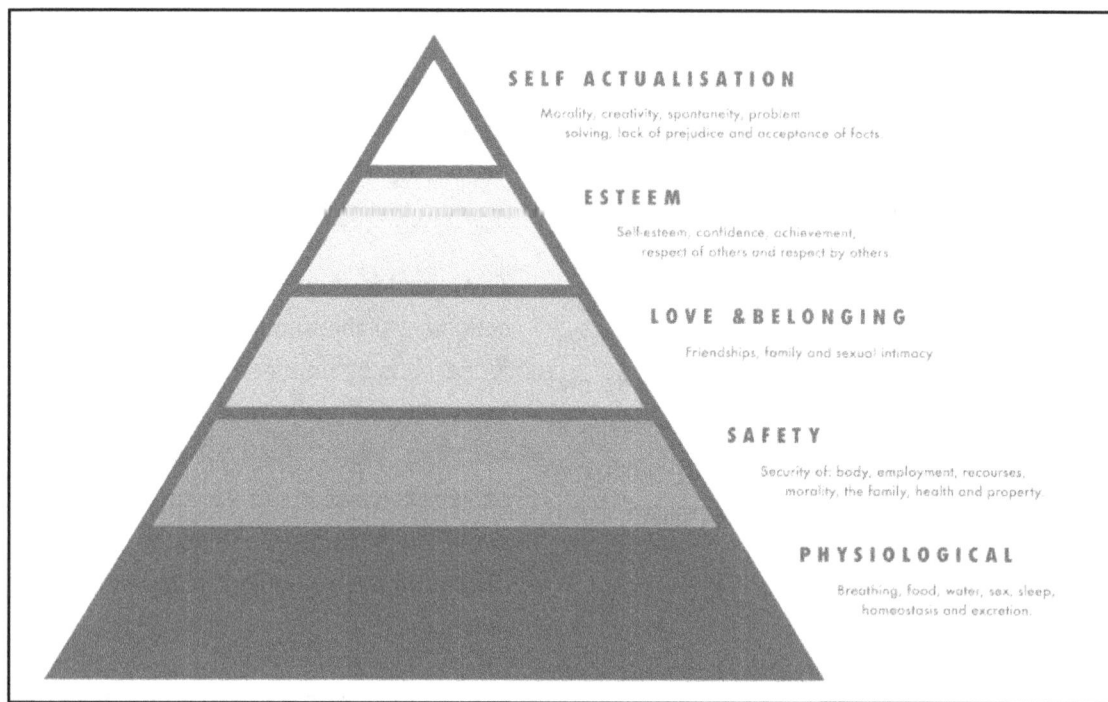

Maslow classified the fifth level of the pyramid as a *growth need* because it enables a person to grow, to reach their full potential as a human being. Once a person has met their deficiency needs, they can turn their attention to self-actualisation. This requires qualities such as honesty, independence, creativity, awareness, objectivity, and originality.

While the theory is generally portrayed as a rigid hierarchy, Maslow noted that the order in which these needs are fulfilled does not always follow a standard progression. For example, he noted that in some individuals, the need for self-esteem is more important than the need for love. For others, the need for creative fulfilment may supersede even basic needs.

Other criticisms of Maslow's theory note that his definition of self-actualisation is difficult to test scientifically. His research on self-actualisation was also based on a very limited sample of individuals, including people he knew as well as biographies of famous individuals that Maslow believed to be self-actualised.

Regardless of these criticisms, Maslow's work represents part of an important shift in psychology. Rather than focusing purely on abnormal behaviour, Maslow's humanistic psychology was focused on the development of healthy individuals. As such it can be a useful model for us to draw ideas from that relate to our own lives.

No model can ever fully represent reality but they can give us a structure through which we can examine our own personal situations. Let's look at the five levels.

Level One: Physiological Needs

The basic physiological needs are fairly apparent, being things vital to our survival. Examples include: food, water, breathing, homeostasis. In addition to these basic requirements, the physiological needs also include such things as shelter and clothing as well as sexual reproduction (being essential to the propagation of the species.)

Level Two: Security and Safety Needs

At the second level, the requirements start to become a bit more complex. The need for security and safety become primary, including: financial security, heath and wellness, safety against accidents and injury. Finding work, getting health care, having savings, are all examples of actions motivated by security and safety needs. These first two levels taken together are termed *basic needs.*

Level Three: Social Needs

The third level includes such things as love, acceptance, and belonging. At this level, the need for emotional relationships drives human behaviour. Some of the things that satisfy this need would include: friendships, romantic attachments, family, social and community groups, churches and religious organizations

In order to avoid problems such as loneliness, depression, and anxiety, it is important for people to feel loved and accepted by others. Personal relationships play an important role here, alongside involvement in religious groups, sports teams, book clubs, and other similar activities.

Level Four: Esteem Needs

The fourth level is the need for appreciation and respect. When the needs at the bottom three levels have been satisfied, esteem needs begin to play a more prominent role in motivating behaviour. People have a need to accomplish things and then have their efforts recognised. People need to sense that they are valued and by others and feel that they are making a contribution to the world.

Participation in professional activities, academic accomplishments, athletic or team participation, and personal hobbies can all play a role in fulfilling esteem needs.

Levels three and four combined are termed *psychological needs.*

Level Five: Self-Actualisation Needs

At the peak of Maslow's hierarchy are the self-actualisation needs. *What a man can be, he must be,* Maslow explained, referring to the need people have to achieve their full potential as human beings. He defined self-actualisation as: *The full use and exploitation of talents, capabilities, potentialities, etc. Such people seem to be fulfilling themselves and to be doing the best that they are capable of doing. They are people who are developing to the full stature of which they capable.*

Self-actualising people are self-aware, concerned with personal growth, less concerned with the opinions of others, and interested in fulfilling their potential.

THE HIERARCHIES AND STRESS

How does this model fit into our work on stress? One way is to use it to pinpoint areas in our lives that may be causing stress or anxiety. Work through each level and make note of areas of your own life you think are lacking on this scale. There may be several areas you can identify. For example, you might want a secure job, a partner and creative fulfilment. The hierarchy allows you to figure out what to focus on first. By handling your job first, you'll create a solid base and reduce your stress. This should put you in a better position to find a partner and, from there to finally focus on being all you can be.

Likewise, we can also use this model to understand and even improve our relationships with others, whether they be domestic or whether they be in the workplace. Understanding other peoples' motivations means that we are better equipped to respond to their needs and so better manage their expectations and activities.

Have you ever been in one of those meetings that drags on and on into lunchtime? Once people start getting hungry, what do you think their primary motivation will be? Are they concentrating on the speaker or are they thinking about a nice cheese roll?

Similarly, imagine being an employee who is never thanked or made to feel appreciated. How would you feel in that situation, how would it effect your morale and willingness to put in extra effort at work?

By understanding the way our brain interprets the world around us, we can gain control over our own and other people's stress and begin to use it to our benefit. Encouragement in the right place will likely lead to increased enthusiasm and output. Stress will only lead to people losing incentive, resulting in lower productivity.

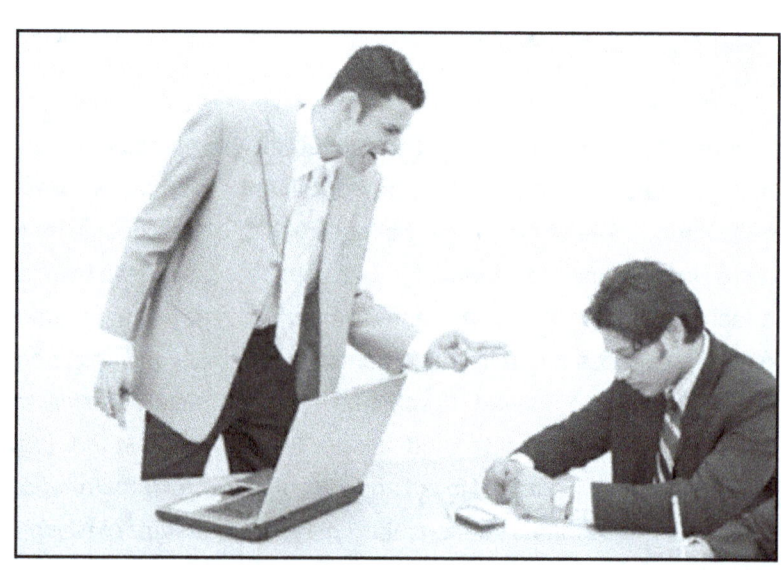

LIFESTYLE REVIEW

If you have been keeping a stress journal and following some of the other suggestion in this book, you have already begun a lifestyle review. However, you may wish to take this further and carry out a more in-depth examination of yourself and your circumstances. This can incorporate as many aspects of your life as you wish - personal, social, financial and so on.

Think of it as taking a snapshot of your life now. This will give you a chance to assess where you are in relation to where you want to be, give you the chance to make relevant changes and allow you to set goals for the future. This might be something you want to make an annual event. Here's some ideas on how to get started

SET ASIDE THE TIME AND PLACE

Give yourself sufficient time to complete the process. You don't have to finish it in one sitting, you might set aside a number of sessions over the course of a week. A good time might be between Christmas and New Year, this is usually a period of downtime for most of us.

Make sure you have suitable surroundings, too. Minimise distractions - no computer or mobile phone! Set up in a comfortable place, have some nice music playing, arm yourself with pen and notebook.

Be honest in your review, try not to miss anything out or exaggerate anything. Work through the procedure, feel free to skip any sections that are not relevant.

STEP 1 MILESTONES

Begin by making a time-line of the year just gone. Add onto it all major milestones and events in that year. Births, marriages, deaths, Changes of job, moving house, relationship situations. Perhaps you completed a course, got a qualification, suffered an illness. All should be added. The chart doesn't have to be detailed, you can make a simple list by month.

STEP 2 EXAMINE

Once finished, sit back and read through your milestones list. When ready, answer the following questions:

What were your two or three biggest accomplishments over the year?
Are there any other goals achieved that you are you proud of?
How did you grow over the past twelve months?
What are some healthy habits you integrated into your life?
What are some new skills you developed?
What were the biggest obstacles you overcame this year?
What were the two or three best decisions you made all year? What did you learn from those experiences?
What risks did you take and what were the rewards?
What were your biggest failures? What did you learn from them?

What were some bad habits you adopted?
What were the two or three worst decisions you made this year? What did you learn from them?
What new relationships enhanced your life? Who? How?
What single person had the biggest impact (positive or negative) on your life? How?
What were the two or three peak moments this year? What were you doing? What did you learn?
What were the two or three lowest moments this year? What happened? What did you learn?
What five to seven words describe this year?
What are you most thankful for?

STEP 3 SATISFACTION SCORES

Copy out the following list of ten topics and assess your satisfaction in each by giving a score from one to ten. One means completely dissatisfied, ten means as good as it can be. Each topic heading is followed by some suggestions as to what you might wish to base your score on.

Health - *energy levels, nutrition, sleep, exercise, mood, general mental state.*
Family / friends - *quality of relationships.*
Love - *romance, connection, intimacy, sex.*
Money - *financial situation, income, expenses, debt and financial freedom.*
Career - *current work career trajectory, work/life balance, co-workers, status.*
Spirituality - *religion, beliefs, rituals, practices, meditations, expression.*
Personal Growth - *self-improvement, creativity, training, learning, coaching.*
Fun - *recreation, travel, hobbies.*
Technology - *time spent on-line, ability to disconnect.*
Environment - *home, living space, country, city / town and workspace.*

The aim is not to score ten in each category, it is to find a balance in your life. This chart will help you see which areas need changes. Look at your scores and ask which areas you want to improve on in the coming year. Choose just two or three in order to maintain focus.

STEP 4 PLAN AHEAD

In this step we define, visualise and plan where we are heading in the year ahead. We can help clarify our goals with some more questions

What three big goals will you accomplish next year? What's important about them?
What two or three new skills will you acquire?
How do you intend to be different by the end of next year?
Who do you want to become?
What do you want or need to drop?
What are two or three habits or behaviours you will stop?
What are two or three habits or behaviours you will start?
How will you step out of your comfort zone and face your fears?

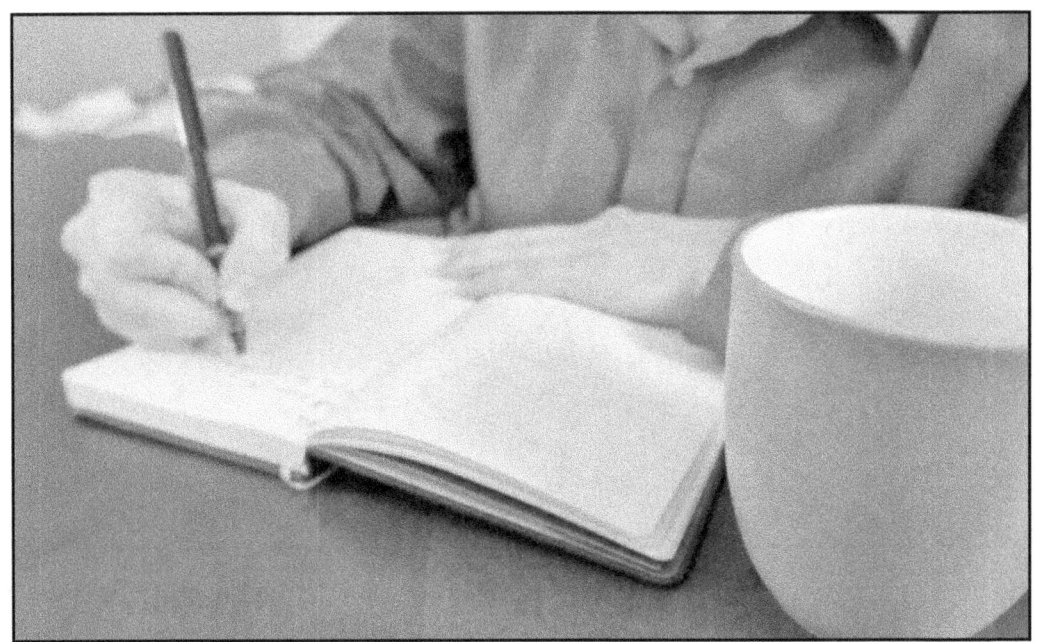

What obstacles will you face and how will you overcome them to accomplish your goals?
Who in your life deserves more attention?
Who do you plan to build a new relationship with?
What are the next steps you can take towards your goals? Be specific!
What resources do you need in order to start making progress?
Who will you seek help from?
How can you evaluate your progress?

That's the complete process. As you can see, it may take a little time and work but by the end you will have a clear picture of where you are and where you are going. Of course, any plans we make will only come to fruition if we follow through on our actions! It might also be useful to conduct monthly "mini-reviews." Get the list out and see if your scores are heading the right way. Adapt as necessary, don't feel you have to be totally locked into any plan - and don't forget, fun and relationships are also on the list. This isn't all about striving for "success" at work to the detriment of everything else. Balance is key!

ACTIVITIES AND THERAPIES

Part of the above plan may well include taking up new activities or seeking out therapies. But where to start and what to choose? Below is a general guide to some of the more common activities that are available, again, all with the caveat of finding a suitably qualified and experienced practitioner. Activities can bring so many benefits, physical, emotional and social. Check out your local area for groups / classes.

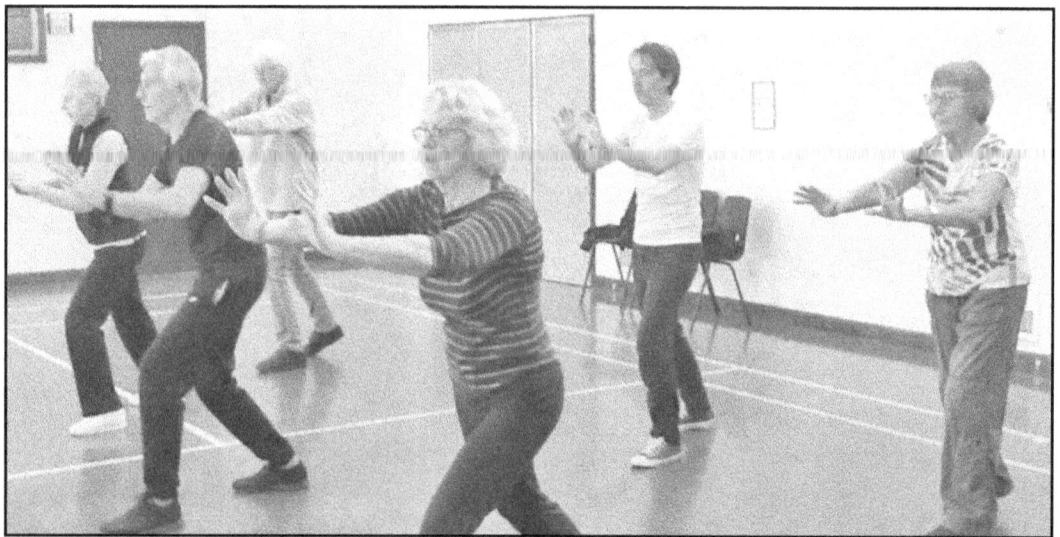

EXERCISE

Even in rural areas there's a wide range of exercise classes to choose from these days. They range from intense cardio workouts through to general fitness classes, yoga and the like. From a stress perspective, I would recommend going for the more mindful forms of exercise. Running on a treadmill will work cardio but we tend not to be mentally involved in the exercise. Activities such as dance, yoga, etc have more of a mind-body balance to them.

MARTIAL ARTS

This covers a very wide range of styles and methods. They can broadly be divided into traditional, sporting and combative arts. Traditional are those system developed over generations, such as the various styles of Kung Fu, Karate and so on. Good traditional styles are usually holistic, in that they also incorporate methods of health, healing and meditation. They may be more or less culturally or combative inclined depending on the emphasis of the particular teacher. Many people practice martial arts purely for the personal benefits, with little or no thought of fighting. Some arts, such as Tai Chi, have become well known as health / mindful practices.

Sporting arts include boxing, MMA, Thai Boxing and so on. They are usually highly structured with a clear syllabus and progression. They are likely to include a high fitness content as well as lots of contact - though some classes have adapted more for fitness, such as boxercise and so on. Sports give you the chance to test your skills in competition.

Combative arts are usually developed for military use, using a mixture of traditional and sporting methods. They may focus less on fitness and more on quick-to-learn self defence techniques. A good school will also focus on awareness, avoidance and fear control. They may offer some of the benefits of traditional arts but without the cultural attachments.

My own personal preference, having trained for decades in martial arts, is the Russian discipline of Systema. If you find a good Systema teacher, you will enjoy an art that covers all aspects of human movement and behaviour, as well as having an in-depth health and well-being aspect.

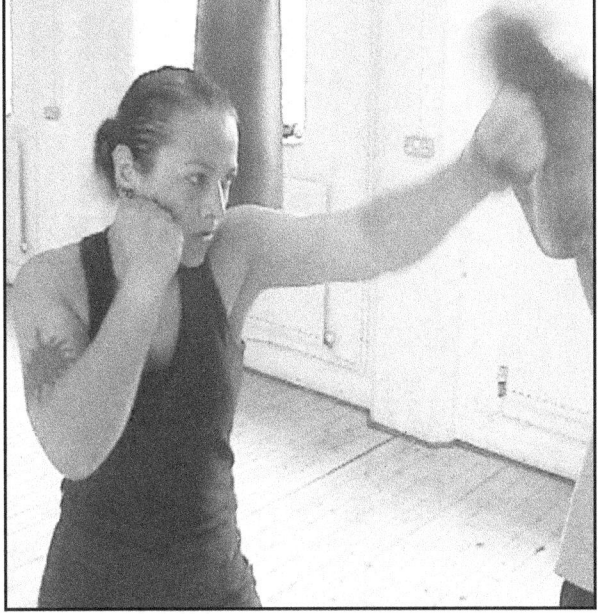

SPIRITUALITY

For generations, humans have asked why are we here, what is the meaning of life and similar questions. For answers, many turn to spirituality, religion, philosophy, art, and nature. Spirituality and its expression are unique to each individual. For some, it is enough to feel a part of nature. For others, it is expressed through the tenets and practices of a formal religion.

Of course, there are also those who decry both and look purely to science for meaning and explanation. Science-vs-religion has become a common field of argument in modern times, though statistics point to the number of people who identify as spiritual as increasing. Research also indicates that people involved in spiritual practices are more likely to live longer, report higher levels of happiness and have a lower risk of depression and suicide. This has been explained by the fact that spiritual people engage in practices known to reduce levels of stress. For example, they are more likely to do voluntary work, practice mediation, have stronger community bonds, turn to faith to deal with difficult emotions and encourage forgiveness.

There are as many approaches to spirituality as the exercise methods we mentioned earlier, so if interested in exploring this subject, where do we begin? Some of the exercises already covered are a good start - our mindful practices help put us in touch with our inner selves. Being out in nature helps our feeling of connection to

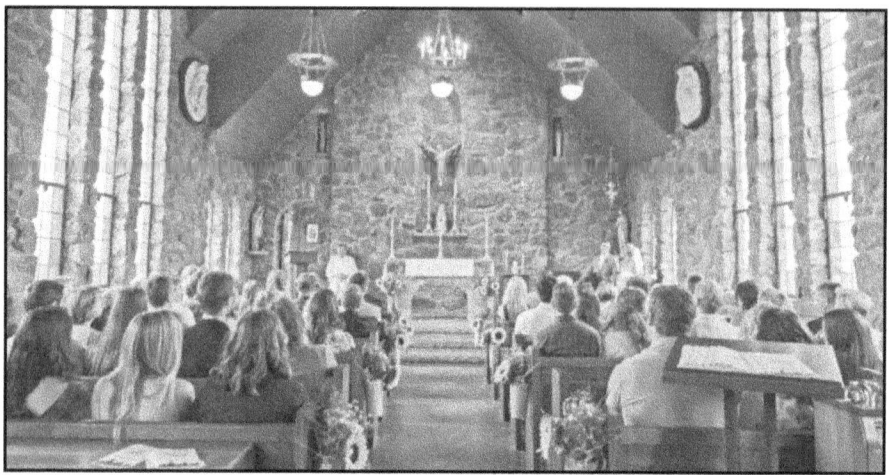

the world at large. You might also look at taking up voluntary work, helping out at a local charity or care home. Doing so can bring us a sense of purpose and positivity, as well as bring perspective and new friends into our life.

Beyond that, think about the type of people that you want to surround yourself with, then join groups and events where you are likely to find them. The same caveats apply as with other activities. Try and find a reputable group, there are unfortunately those willing to take advantage of the emotionally vulnerable and draw them into unhealthy relationships. Don't fall for promise of "unicorns and rainbows," be aware that true spirituality often means facing up to some of the harder questions of life. Let your intuition be your guide and listen to friends and family.

THERAPIES

Most stress-based therapies revolve around having a regular meeting with a counsellor and talking through your issues. A good counsellor will create a safe space, where you feel at ease in discussing your experiences and feelings without judgement. Even just talking to someone can help. In the UK, it was discovered that having a GP spend a little more time talking to patients helps dramatically with well being.

A counsellor will have a structured approach, depending their particular discipline, to lead you through a healing process. That may involve just talking, on your own or with your partner. Hypnotherapy involves putting a person into a deep trance in order to influence behaviour patterns. Cognitive Behavioural Therapy is another method of changing negative patterns and teaching how to regulate our emotions. Behavioural Activation is a talking therapy that aims to help people with depression take simple steps towards enjoying life again.

Art therapy is a form of psychotherapy which

uses the creative process of making art to explore issues and emotions which may be too difficult to express in words. It can also be used to relieve stress and improve mental well-being. Art therapy can include drawing, painting, photography and modelling.

There are also many group therapies available, from support groups to groups teaching new skills. Group work can be very beneficial in dealing with addiction issues, they can also bring a social aspect to the therapy which may also be useful.

Therapies may combined with other activities as part of an overall well-being package. Doctors now recognise the positive mental effects of physical activity as well the more traditional talking methods.

MEDICATION

There are an increasingly wide range of drugs available to treat various mental conditions. This has an up and a down side. On the positive side, a short course of drugs may lift a person out of immediate depression, give them a chance to "reset" and get into therapy. On the downside, places like the USA now have an increasing "opiod crisis" with people becoming addicted to legal drugs. We have seen the same in the past with drugs such as Valium, where popping a pill becomes the answer to any problem. The trouble is that this tends to achieve nothing but masking the problem or

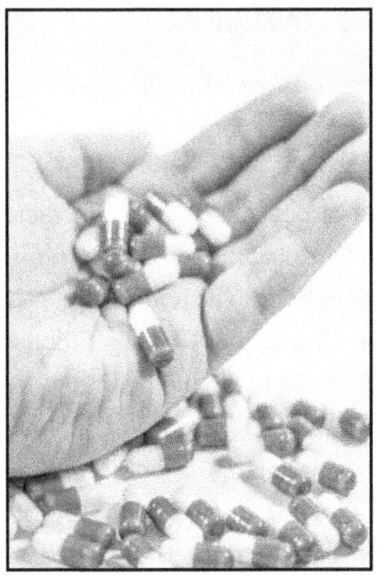

numbing us from its effects. The underlying issues remain unresolved, leading is into that downward spiral we spoke about before.

Obviously, always work under medical advice but be wary of medication becoming a habit. It is a short term measure, at best. Also be aware that there may be more natural or less harmful alternatives to pharmaceuticals - herbal remedies, essential oils and so on. As with everything, do your research first.

We will finish the book with three exercises that are more advanced versions of some of our earlier methods. Other than extra time, they require nothing more than a quiet environment and a strong mental focus. Like anything, these exercises get easier with practice and after a while you will find you can almost have them running in the background during any quiet time.

PULSE BREATHING

This exercise takes us a little deeper into our internal system. Before trying this, it is good to have some experience in the Selective Tension exercise we described earlier. In fact, if you have the time, it is a good idea to run through that exercise prior to doing this one.

Pulse Breathing means consciously connecting our breath and heart rate together. The first step is being able to feel your pulse, At first, we do this using one of the methods below. Later, you will be able to feel your pulse in different parts of the body on an internal level.

FEELING THE PULSE

The sensation of a pulse is, of course, the result of the heart beating and circulating blood around the body. The pulse rate is the number of beats the heart makes per minute. A normal heart rate should be somewhere between 60 to 100 beats per minute, but it can go up to 130–150 beats per minute when exercising. The two most common methods of feeling the pulse are:

Radial pulse
Accesses the radial artery at the wrist.
Place index and middle fingers on the inside of your opposite wrist just below the thumb.

Carotid pulse
Accesses the carotid artery in the neck.
Place index and middle fingers on the side of your windpipe just below the jawbone.

If you wish, you can count the pulses you feel for 15 seconds, then multiply this number by 4 to obtain your heart rate.

To begin with, access your pulse using one of the above methods. Establish a comfortable breathing rhythm using Circular Breathing - eg, inhale for three, exhale for three.

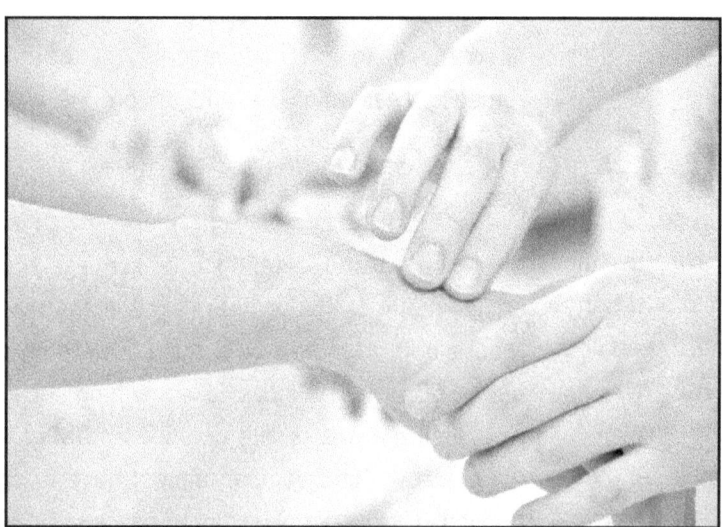

Once you can feel the pulse with the fingers, next work to feel it purely as an internal sensation. If you find this difficult, try doing a few minutes exercise to elevate your pulse - such as squat-thrusts or short sprints. Then sit or stand quietly, you should be able to feel a strong pulse in different parts of the body.

In the full exercise, we work around different sections of the body in sequence, feeling the pulse in each. When ready, lay in a quiet place, on your back with arms at your sides. Work into Circular Breathing - you may wish to add in a couple of minutes Wave or Selective Tension here.

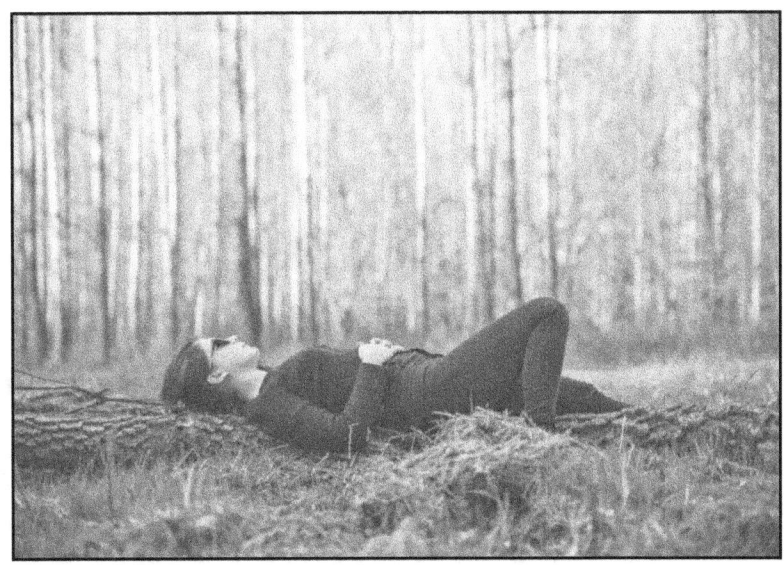

Start by feeling the pulse in your temples. Focus only on the sensation in that area. From there, we work down the body, you can try the suggested order below.

Temples
Neck
Heart
Upper Arms
Hands
Stomach
Groin
Knees
Feet

Once completed, work to bring all those individual areas together into one unified pulse that moves through the whole body. Again, you can work to synchronise breathing and heart beat if you wish, in whichever way is most comfortable.

To finish, let the pulse feeling fade away and return the focus to just the breathing. When ready, slowly stretch and move around a little, then sit up.

You may find it easier to feel the pulse in some places than in others. However with practice, you will soon be able to tap easily into the pulse. Advanced practitioners can slow the heart rate through slowing the breathing, a powerful method of dealing with stress.

As always, should you feel any detrimental effects then come out of the drill immediately. Remember, this is a relaxed exercise so don't try and force anything.

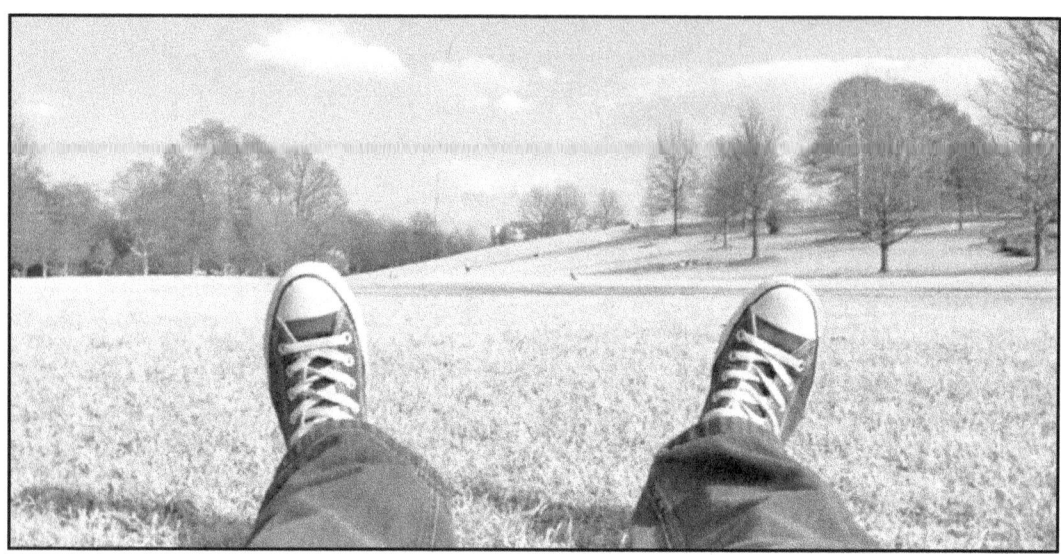

EXTENDED QUIET SITTING

This version of the exercise aims to involve all of our senses, building a connection between the outside world and our internal state. It is best to practice outdoors if you can - perhaps your garden, if it is private, or a quiet spot, somewhere you will not be disturbed.

Lay down and close your eyes. Begin Circular Breathing, slowing your breath and letting the body relax. Run through the Selective Tension exercise, each muscle group in turn, inhale tense, exhale relax. Once you have worked round all the muscles, inhale and tense from head to toe, exhale relax three times.

Go back into Circular Breathing. Feel your body relax and sink into the ground. Be aware of the sensation. Notice the air around you, the breeze on your skin, the feel of the sun on your face.

Keep your eyes closed and focus on what you can hear. The wind in the trees, distant traffic, birdsong. Examine each sound in turn, then let them all meld into one.

After a while, on an inhalation, pick up on the scents around you. Flowers, wood smoke, ozone. Again, take each one in turn then let them all meld.

Next, start to move your body a little, twist and stretch. When ready, slowly sit up and open your eyes. Look down at the patch of ground immediately in front of you. Choose something there, a plant, a blade of grass, and study it for a few minutes. Notice its shape, its colour, how it moves. Does it have a scent?

Now, expand your vision out to the wider patch of ground before you and notice all the things there - plants, insects and so on. Watch them, listen to them them, smell them.

After that, raise your eyes and begin to widen out your gaze. Start with what is close to you, trees, bushes, etc then slowly expand out, forward and sideways, into middle and far vision. Do the same with your hearing and smell, try and pick up as much information as you can. Keep an awareness of the sensations in your body - your contact with the ground, your posture, your breathing.

Next, switch between that far vision and the near object you first looked at. Once you've done this for a while, finish by slowly standing, then stretch and move a little, but all the while maintaining that outward connection. Walk around and touch some of the things you have been looking at. Hug a tree, it's a nice feeling!

TAI CHI MINDFUL MOVEMENT

Traditional Tai Chi routines (called forms) are made up of around 108 movements, performed in a slow, continual flow. They take around 15-20 minutes to perform and can be quite physically and mentally demanding.

For our purposes, in order to practice some mindful movement, we will look at the very first of the Tai Chi form, called Lift Hands. This is one of the more straightforward moves, so is very easy to learn. Having said that, there are many layers that can be added in to even the most simple postures in Tai Chi - including structure, breathing patterns, spiral movement and so on but we will stick to the basics here.

Our start posture is to stand in a comfortable,

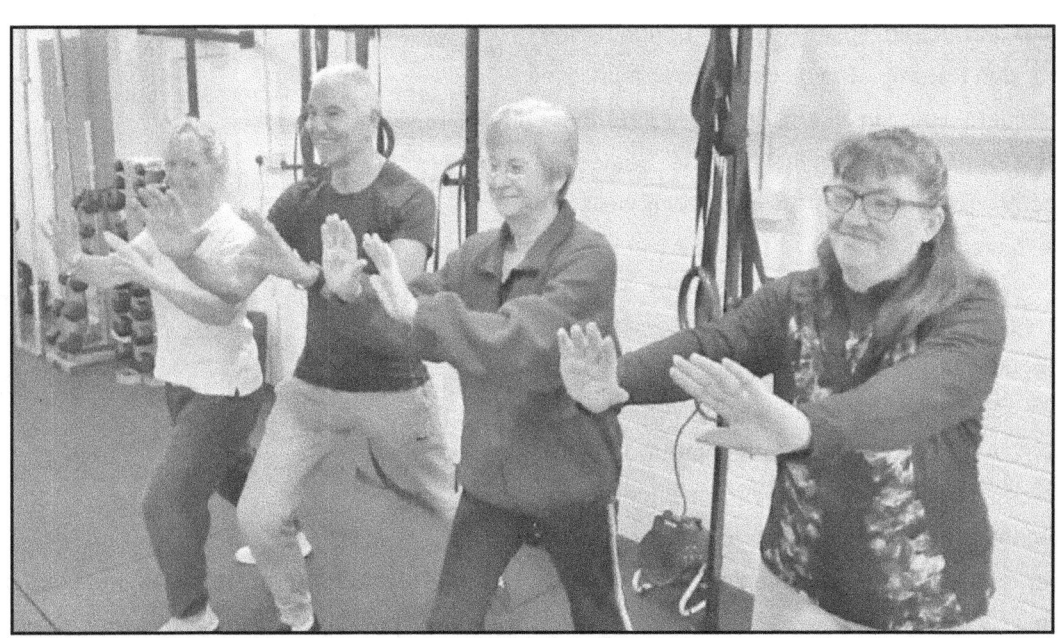

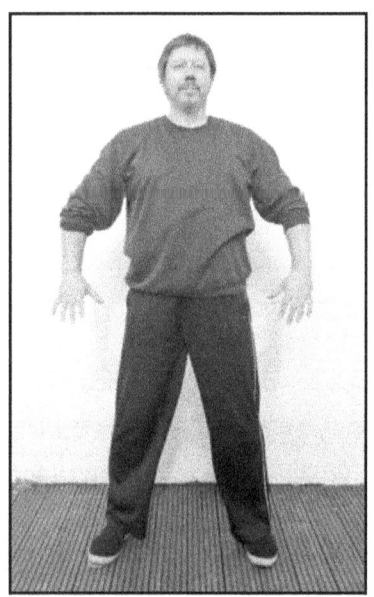 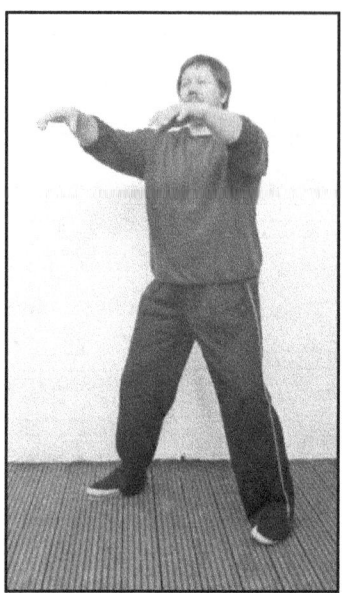 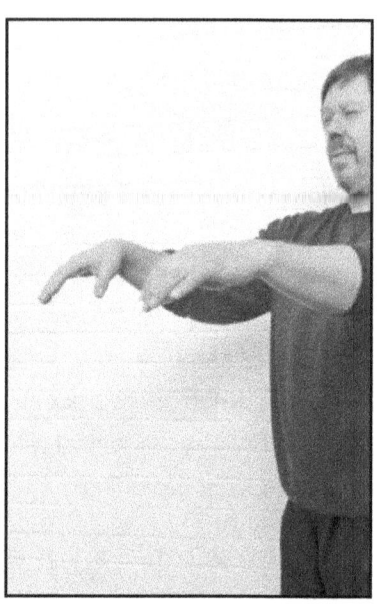

upright position, with the feet close together. The arms hang at the sides, keeping the armpits open, the palms facing back.

Spend a minute or in this posture, focus on your breathing and allow the body to relax and settle. Relax but not collapse! Keep an upright spine and don't slump. If you feel tension in the shoulders, you can lift and drop, or rotate them a few times to get rid of the stiffness. Settle into Circular Breathing. On an inhalation, we start the movement.

Sink all your weight into the left leg. Raise the right heel and draw a semi-circle with your right toes, taking the foot out to a little over shoulder width. As you do that the arms open out a little more to the side. As you exhale, the fingers point forward and the palms press down towards the floor. You sink the weight evenly in the feet, what is called a 50-50 stance.

Now, as you inhale, slowly raise the hands up to shoulder height. Actually don't raise them, it is better if you think of them as "floating" up. This is one of the characteristics of Tai Chi movement. To lift the hands, most people engage the shoulders but this brings tension. Instead, imagine you are standing in deep water. Your feet sink into the sand but your body is supported by the water, your arms feel light. Let the water lift your hands, they feel weightless.

You might also imagine you are a puppet, your body is suspended from above by a string through the crown of the head. Another string is attached to each wrist and it is these that raises the hands. As the arms raise, the wrists and fingers relax, sinking down a little as shown in the picture above.

On the exhale, the arms slowly lower back to the start position. As the hands lower, the wrists

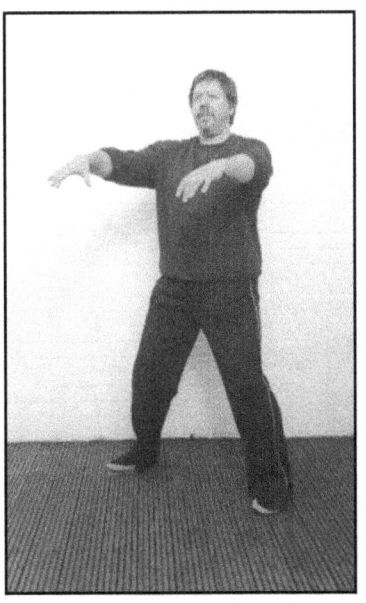 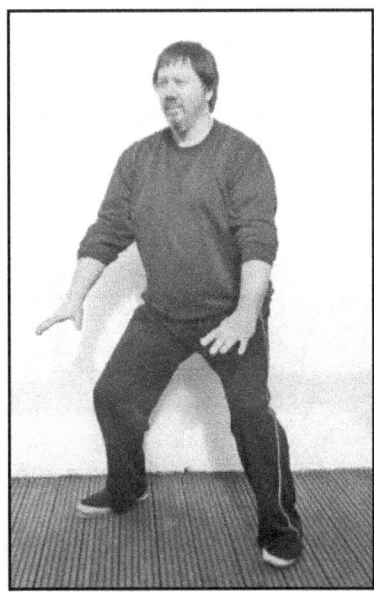 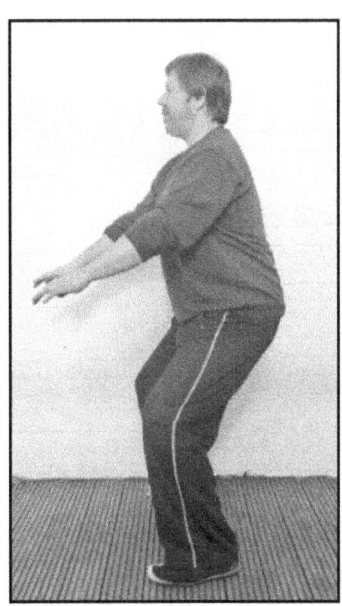

flex a little, allowing the fingers to lift up. The action should be like you are painting with a large brush, sweeping up, sweeping down.

As the hands lower, you can also sink down a little into your legs. No need to go into a full squat, just go as low as you are comfortable with. Be sure that you are keeping the spine straight, particularly the lower back. It is okay to lean a little, but keep the spine as straight as you can. Also check that your knees do not collapse in as you sink - you can turn the toes out a little if it helps.

As far as the breathing goes, you should co-ordinate the speed of your in hale / exhale with the rise and fall of the hands. Slow the breath a little and keep movement and breathing smooth and even. This is one facet of mindfulness within the Tai Chi moves - working both internal and external aspects. Once used to the movement, you can add in an expansion of the rib cage on the lift/inhale and a relaxation of the chest on the sink/exhale. From there, you can work into diaphragmatic breathing if you wish.

Take your time with all of this, do not rush. As the hands lower, try to get a sense of the weight sinking through the soles of the feet and into the ground. Try the movement, repeat it maybe a dozen times or so, that's all you need do at this stage.

So there it is, a simple move but already you can see how many things are involved! This is one reason Tai Chi is preformed slowly most of the time, to allow you to focus on all the requirements of the posture, to add in all the different layers of movement and mental intent. It is this focus that ties our body and mind together, so bringing us firmly into the present moment and letting our worries drift away.

CHAPTER TEN
CONCLUSIONS

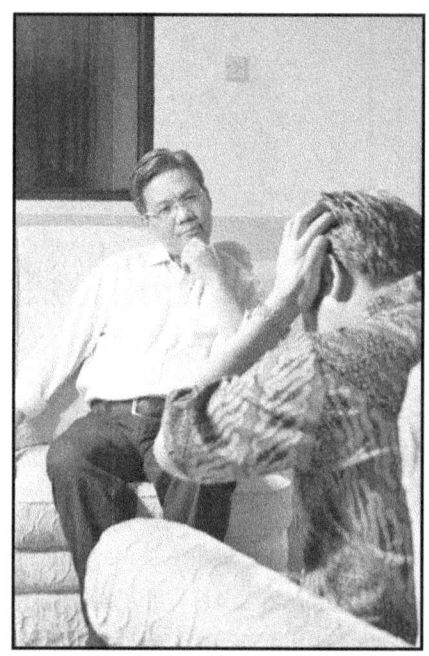

I hope you have found the suggestions in this book useful. If nothing else, I hope you have learnt that while stress is a natural part of life, it is not necessary to give in to it, to allow it to overwhelm us or to feel we are "failures" because we are stressed.

I hope you have also learnt that we don't have to tolerate bad behaviour from other people, and also that it is okay to express our own emotions and feelings. We have the right to be angry, sad, emotional, happy, joyful or down. Expressing our feelings in an appropriate way is healthy, it is cathartic. It is also okay to ask for help, be it personal or professional. There is no need to suffer in silence, no one gets points for "toughing things out." It doesn't mean you have to fold at every minor incident but it does mean you learn to recognise patterns in your behaviour and take charge of them.

Whatever its causes, stress is largely a product of our minds, a reaction to events that have happened or may yet happen. Managing our mental response is the fundamental method of managing stress and tension. The exercises here will give you a good starting point for any further, deeper therapy. If all the exercises appear a bit over-whelming to start, then take things step by step.

I recommend starting with some of the simple breathing exercises, then working into the physical tension drills. From there, try one other method - keeping a journal, perhaps - and see how you go from there. No-one expects you to put all of the suggestions in this book into action at once! Part of managing stress is learning about expectations and finding the right balance of demand and achievement for ourselves.

Think of the process as a marathon rather than a sprint. Most of these methods can, and should, be practiced well into old age - stress doesn't lessen with time, we always have to keep our defences up!

Aside from the breathing exercises, the single most powerful thing you can do to manage your stress is to be in control of your mindset. As much as possible, learn to live in the here and now. This is what experts call the *Flow State* - the place that sports people, martial artists and musicians strive to be, where everything becomes effortless and full of joy.

It is unrealistic to expect ourselves to be in that state constantly - we have to think about the future and reflect on the past at some point! But when carrying out everyday tasks, or when pressures begin to mount, always try and keep your focus on the now, on the moment. Appreciate the small things in life, the fresh air, the warm sun or the cold rain! Be mindful in your activities.

The digital world is very good at pulling us out of that state and into the virtual world, often at the expense of interactions in the real world. Consider limiting your on-line time, or even try a digital detox. Perhaps you could set aside a set time every week for a purely *you* activity.

Simply Flow

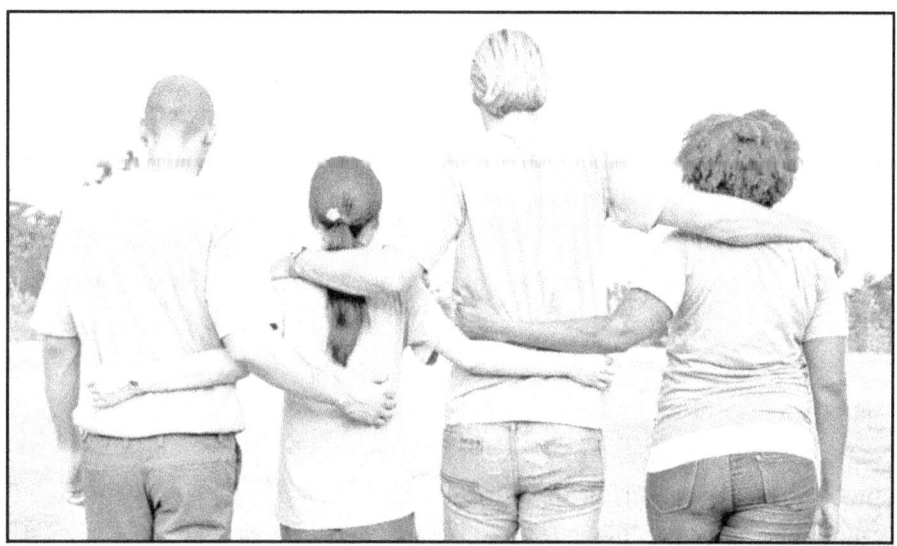

Turn off your PC and phone for an hour, just sit and read a book, for example.

Alternatively, put aside some time to help others - an elderly neighbour, perhaps. The second most powerful method of dealing with stress is having a good community around you, be it friends, family or other support. You don't have to deal with any problems alone!

I also hope this book will make you more aware of stress in other people. Learn to recognise the signs, even though people may try and hide the fact they are having problems. Sometimes people channel their stress into anger or aggression, or into destructive behaviour. If you see this happening, try to understand the root cause of the problem and see if you can help the person appropriately.

Of course, not everyone welcomes help. People might see it as interfering, they may be in denial over their issues. They may feel that being stressed shows weakness of character, or may be too proud to ask for help, so always temper your approach accordingly.

It is hard to envision a stress-free world. Perhaps there will come a time when we can conquer disease, starvation and all the other ills that beset us. Even then, it is difficult to imagine a world without arguments, relationship issues or similar worries! But by accepting that stress will enter our lives, we can begin to take all the steps we need to manage it, or even to use it to our advantage in some circumstances. There is no need to over-complicate issues, even the most complex cases can usually be boiled down to a few simple choices - and we almost always have a choice. So choose to live your life the way you want to live it.

Don't worry. Be happy!

STRESS MANAGEMENT CHECKLIST

IMMEDIATE STRESS

- Burst / Circle Breathing
- Remain calm and take appropriate action
- If in danger of harm, remove yourself from situation where possible

POST - EVENT STRESS

- Movement to dispel tension or as tension begins
- Quiet Sitting to calm nerves

PRE-EVENT STRESS

- Preparation
- Breathing to control nerves

STRATEGIES

- Stress trigger journal
- Compensation journal
- Review your coping mechanisms
- Conduct an annual lifestyle review

LIFESTYLE

- Eat a balanced diet
- Make sure you are getting enough sleep
- Monitor life-work balance
- Do you need to say *No* more?
- Get appropriate support and help where necessary

LONG TERM

- Take up mindful exercise
- Set aside quiet time for breathing/meditation, massage, etc
- Try new hobbies or learning
- Build up a support network
- Adjust your mindset

Simply Flow

Don't Worry!

APPENDIX ONE

MP3 DOWNLOADS

If you go to the link below, you will find a number of MP3 files that you can download. Each file will talk you through one of the various selective tension or visualisation exercises. Once in your comfortable position, simply play the track on your player / headphones and follow the instructions.

http://www.mediafire.com/folder/yd6dtvaq0l10l/STRESS_MP3s

Simply Flow

APPENDIX TWO

RESOURCES

This list is by no means exhaustive but includes some of the main organisations that provide support and help.

GENERAL HELP

SAMARITANS www.samaritans.org   Call 116 123 24/7

MIND MENTAL HEALTH   www.mind.org.uk

CITIZENS ADVICE BUREAU   www.citizensadvice.org.uk

DEBT ADVICE   www.nationaldebtline.org

CHILDLINE   www.childline.org.uk

SHOUT   www.giveusashout.org

AGE UK   www.ageuk.org.uk

COUNSELLING & SUPPORT SERVICES

NHS   www.nhs.uk/conditions/counselling

RELATE   www.relate.org.uk

ALCOHOLICS ANONYMOUS   www.alcoholics-anonymous.org.uk

ACTION ON ADDICTION   www.actiononaddiction.org.uk

SUPPORTLINE   www.supportline.org.uk

BRITISH COUNSELLING ASSOCIATION   www.bacp.co.uk

HYPNOTHERAPY DIRECTORY   www.hypnotherapy-directory.org.uk

BRITISH PSYCHOLOGICAL SOCIETY   www.bps.org.uk

NATIONAL COUNSELLING SOCIETY   www.nationalcounsellingsociety.org

BEREAVEMENT CARE   www.cruse.org.uk

Simply Flow

APPENDIX THREE

CONTACT DETAILS

E-MAIL   simplyflow@outlook.com

WEBSITE   www.simplyflow.co.uk

FACEBOOK GROUP www.facebook.com/groups/sflow/

SHOP SITE   www.systemafilms.com

Sign up to our mailing list for news and offers   http://eepurl.com/dmNQhz

SYSTEMA   www.russianmartialart.com

If you have enjoyed this book, please leave us a
review on Amazon.
Thanks!

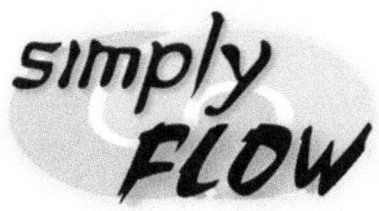

NOTES

NOTES

EIGHT BROCADES QIGONG

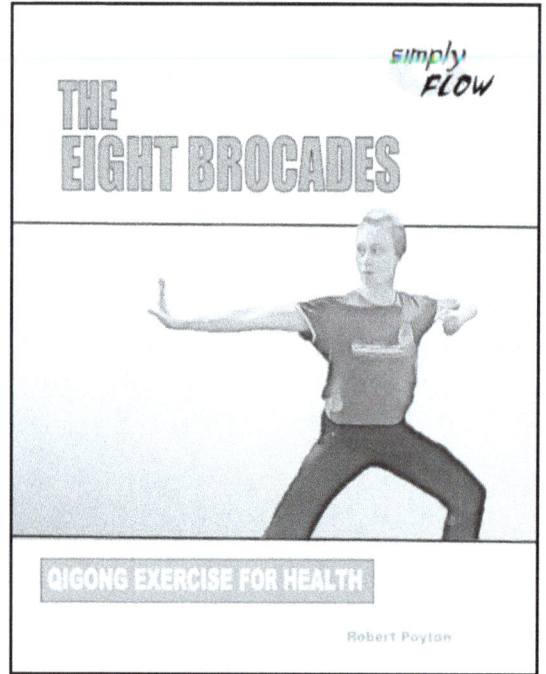

Qigong or Chi Kung is an umbrella term for many forms of Chinese exercise. Whether for health, fitness, meditation or martial arts, qigong methods have been developed over hundreds of years.

The Eight Brocades are a very popular set of qigong exercises. Comprising of eight simple movements, they provide a good, all-round gentle body workout. However there is more to qigong than twisting and stretching!

The movements also combine with specific breathing patterns and visualisations to work the body's internal systems. This also means they are a very good method for improving health, dealing with stress and developing mindfulness.

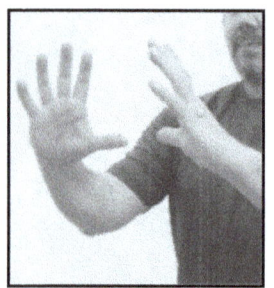
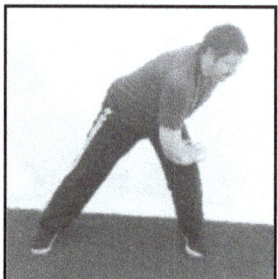

In this book, experienced Instructor Robert Poyton teaches you the complete Eight Brocades routine, plus some variations. He also details the historical background of the Eight Brocades and explains the basics of Traditional Chinese Medicine.

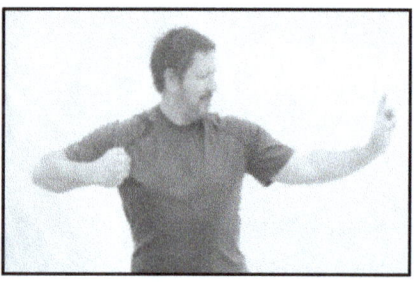

Requiring little space and easily adjusted to fit your personal circumstances, the Eight Brocades are a great routine for anyone looking to improve their health and well-being

Paperback / PDF   100 pages

FITNESS OVER 40

Many people ask how they can maintain health and fitness as they age. Gyms can be expensive and intimidating and many exercise programs focus solely on superficial looks.

The *Simply Flow* Program is all about regaining your body's natural movement, building core strength, boosting your health and learning to manage stress and tension.

It involves simple to learn exercises that easily fit into and enhance all your other activities, as well as giving you a unique Formula to develop your own exercise variations. This book covers all the foundation exercises of the Program, including -

Breathing
Core Strength
Joint Mobility
Stretching
Movement Chains
Resistance Training
Ground Movement
Mindfulness and Flow

Plus advice on diet, lifestyle, developing your own training routines and more.

Looking for a sensible long term exercise program that fits in with and enhances your lifestyle and activities?
Here it is!

Paperback / PDF   126 pages

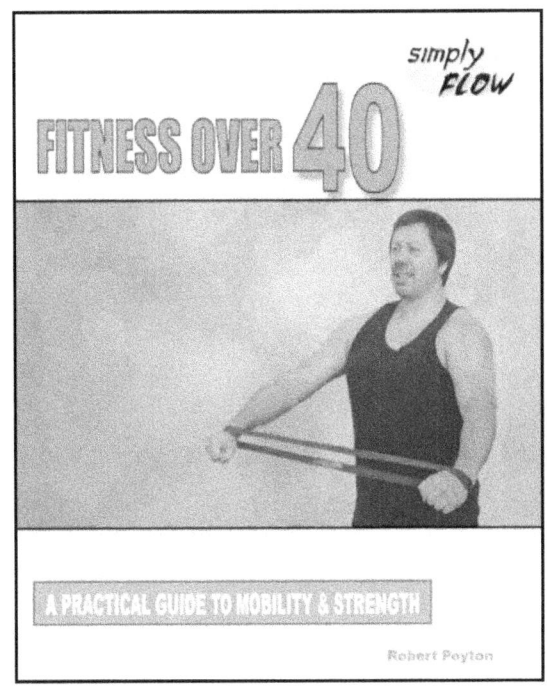

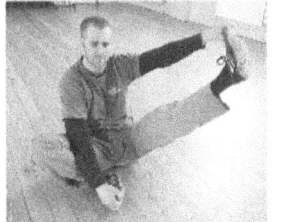 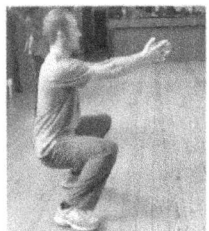

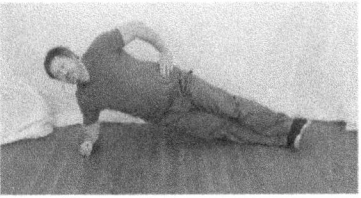

Both books available via Amazon or direct from

www.simplyflow.co.uk

www.ingramcontent.com/pod-product-compliance
Lightning Source LLC
Chambersburg PA
CBHW081110080526
44587CB00021B/3537